JU.

kids need care

Nutrition, Natural Remedies,
and Life-Guidance

Home Media

Printed in the United States of America

First Edition

ISBN: 9781931078344

Cover & book design by Robert Masheris

Disclaimer: This book is not intended as a substitute for medical diagnosis or treatment. Anyone who has a serious disease should consult a physician before initiating any change in treatment or before beginning any new treatment.

For more information call: 1-800-243-5242

For further inquiries send a SASE to:
Home Media
Box 4885
Buffalo Grove, IL 60089

kids
need
care

Foreword

If you are a typical parent trying to give your child the very best, *Kids Need Care* by Judy Gray is an absolute must.

Typical daily excessive chemical exposure and electromagnetic radiation can harm the eggs and sperm of women and men. These exposures can impair the development of infants from the moment of conception, and the harm can last throughout their lives. Surprisingly, it is even possible for the damage to persist through future generations!

The aim must be to lovingly guide and mold all youngsters so they become all they can be. They need to develop into caring exemplary human beings with sensible priorities and lofty values that will manifest in some way during their lives to make our world a better place. They must be nurtured, so they mature and develop to their fullest potential, not only physically but also mentally, emotionally, and spiritually. Each aspect of this is discussed in this book.

There is no way a developing child can manage in this present world without markedly improved nutrition. This book is certainly much more than foods and diets. It contains one fascinating tip about nutrients after another. There are enticing, sensible recipes to tempt your children to eat healthier diets. There is even a sense of urgency because of the extreme neglect of our world for so many decades.

Because of pollution much of our water, air, and food, as well as our homes, schools, and workplaces, are now less healthy than they were in the past. We simply must build up our nutrition and immune defense systems so children and their families can handle the daily onslaught of unavoidable environmental assaults.

Kids Need Care is truly a "how to" book for parents who want to do and be the best.

Doris Rapp, M.D.

Contents

Introduction

These words came together while on a working trip above the 55th parallel. This is an incredible remote northern location far from what many consider to be civilization. It's a place where paved roads end and hard work begins to find the bounty of nature. This isolated area provides a rich array of wilderness medicines and a treasure trove of wild plants and berries. Unfortunately, very few people take advantage of these gifts of nature, including those who live in the area. Most are not even aware of the abundance of nature, let alone the powerful effects of the wild forage. Thus, among many of the men, women, and children—even in the peace of the wilderness communities—their physical, mental, and spiritual health suffer the consequences of depending solely on the man-made realm of chemicals and processed foods even though they are surrounded by the glorious beauty and power of the productive boreal forests. These ancient boreal forests are a fine example of the wild, native, slow-growing trees and foliage and the amazing plant life of the far North. Sadly, the local people there readily accept all the modern practices, food, and drink, which may harm and even destroy their health, wealth, and mental well-being. The answers for a better and stronger life are so near, yet, so distant, because they are largely ignored or rebuffed. The old ways of surviving off the land are considered to be silly or too much work.

The boreal forest endures the direst of extremes. During the long winter light is scarce, and the days and nights are bitterly cold. In the winter months the temperature hovers somewhere above or below -40°C (-40°F). During the short, two-month summer the thermometer may read 40°C (104°F) or above. Because of these extremes the plants and creatures must be strong and resilient if they are to survive. Everything in the wilderness has to work and fight to survive. The top soil, while not too deep, is untouched and, thus, rich in minerals. Therefore, the very texture, color, substance, and appearance of the plants that provide the berries and herbage are superior to any which are commonly found in the polluted and highly populated areas. Cultivated plants, even the organic ones, are inferior to such mighty persistence of this wild flora. Thus, these magnificent wild plants also provide highly unusual nourishment for needy bodies.

The night is slow in coming this far north during the summer months. It is light until 10:00 p.m., even as fall approaches. So, for the wild harvester this allows a lot of picking time. It is slow, backbreaking work in the deep bush with lots of mosquitoes and other biting creatures, not to mention the local fauna such as the bear in their forest home. It is only wise to respect the forest and its creatures. A portion of the wild berries must be left for them to eat, and it is mandatory to leave quickly and quietly if the bear appear threatened or aggressive.

It is also important to be caring of the forest itself. Harvesters take garbage bags as part of the equipment for disposal of refuse left behind by those who are ignorant of maintaining a pristine environment or just don't care. It is vital to never damage the forest vegetation. The wild fruit must survive to be food for all the creatures and to be the main substance in raw, wild berry formulas. The formulas are beneficial for restoring the well-being of so many. Most of them even taste good. However, like the lessons of life, some of the plant medicine is rather bitter, especially some of the wild greens. Yet, like the many lessons that are a part of life on this planet, these wild substances enhance strength and even offer a means of survival.

When the conditions are fairly stable, the animals in these wild places seem to actively reproduce. Their lives are so fragile that nature makes sure that few babies exist or survive when the conditions are most adverse. However, it seems to be a fairly common human custom to give more thought to what's for dinner than to the obligations that exist with bringing a child into the world. Many people take it for granted that children will be in the picture of their lives, but then they never give this event another thought.

In some poor countries children are considered to be part of the personal wealth, perhaps their only wealth. Yet, so many people fail to realize how truly serious the responsibility is to be the caretaker and protector of tiny beings in a world with far too many problems. The family plays a major role in shaping the character of the child. The community environment plus the care and training given at home are the foundation of a child's world. Thus, there should, perhaps, be more focus on teaching children why they are really here. That means they are taught to advance their souls in the finest ways for the greatest good. Of course, every child is a unique soul, and he/she must be accepted and dealt with as an individual.

In this time of great corruption, hate, uncertainty, and war the only things that can stop this downward spiral are upright thoughts. By upright thoughts this means personally achieving and teaching others to seek the highest goals possible without negativity. It is possible to focus on bringing all thoughts and, thus, our lives to the highest levels no matter what the rest of humanity is doing. Each chapter in the book discusses how these thoughts can develop into goals and practices and the methods best employed not only for personal benefit, but also for the benefit of others and the earth itself.

Planet Earth could well be called the University of Life. Everyone will win some events and issues and also lose some. If more are lost than won, then this is a life out of balance. To determine the cause of this an individual must search within. Unfortunately, many people deny that they could be at fault in any way. Until such people let go of this denial habit and the strong negative emotions that accompany such behavior, a balanced life can never be achieved. This eventually leads to disease and one disaster after another.

Every living human experiences a variety of emotions. Some people are more emotional than others, while others lack the finer, kinder, caring emotions. Emotions are the key difference between human and animal behavior. The finest emotions provide the power to evolve into a higher and better state. The negative emotions only bring disaster. Everything depends on the choices made. However, bad choices frequently provide the greatest and longest lasting learning experiences. Of course, these lessons are learned only when the mind is open and ready to receive the messages provided by the experiences.

It is true that every person has different attitudes, abilities, and skills. Likewise, all people are blessed with a single or many talents. Some develop their talents, while others make excuses. Some come into the world with great advantages, which they fail to use humanely, and they ruthlessly exploit others. Then, there are those who are born with few advantages and, despite this, develop miraculously. Some will create joy and happiness among the human condition, while others will create bombs, war, murder, and hate. Some always build, while others continuously destroy. This has not changed during the course of human civilization, and yet, it is a fact that every person writes his/her own history. What's more, it is possible to help others write glowing personal histories of their own. No doubt, this is absolutely the path that is most desirable.

Only a few people will be remembered and noted in the history books. Yet, the lives an individual touches and any fine energy that is activated will be noted in this realm and beyond. It is a personal obligation to do the best that is possible, to refuse to worry about the past and the future, and to build the "present" one day at a time. The present is the only time in which anyone actually lives. The past is over, and there is no rewind button on life experiences. You can only learn from life and never change what is in the past. The future is waiting to exist. Therefore, no one should worry and agitate about either the past or the future. Every day is the "present". It truly is a present—a gift, but only if the choice is to make it so.

The past, present, and future are governed by thoughts. Nothing is impossible, unless it is thought to be so. Could someone eat an elephant? Not that most people would ever want to eat an entire elephant, but if the mind set was to do so, it could happen. It would take a long time, but it could be done—one bite at a time. This rather unlikely example merely means that little to nothing is impossible if you focus, believe with all your heart, and work at it as hard as you can with no negative thoughts of failure. Negative thoughts and worries can only impede or destroy the success that one aspires to achieve.

Thoughts are the most important tools in the human armamentarium. When life isn't going well, take the time to check for negative thoughts. Then, be brutally honest about all personal actions and thoughts. Make a list of any problems, and write out all personal thoughts that pertain to them. In other words, describe on paper what the problems are and what personal contributions may have occurred to cause the problems to exist. Then, are others always to blame for any difficulties? If so, write the reasons for this thinking. Explain in detail what is likely to solve the problems. Don't just write down comments like "lots of money" or "someone needs to help me." Spell out potential solutions that can be personally achieved. Some things may take a long time to sort out, but the above exercise is a start on the right path. It is a helpful tool to think through life experiences and, thus, make better decisions. As confidence increases more successful decisions are achieved. This further leads to being better equipped to lead a powerful life, and it supports individual ability to guide children in the family to their highest potential.

It is important to be aware of the potential and needs of each child. This helps in making better decisions concerning every child's welfare and to be prepared to lovingly guide him/her. Children are like blank sheets of paper, and they must be taught how to think most effectively and make appropriate decisions. Most children can do anything exceedingly well that corresponds with their innate talents and desires. Yet, they can learn and do countless other skills and disciplines which they think they may not even like.

Consider what happens if individual talents are not recognized. Most adults wrongly pursue what they think will make money instead of identifying their true talents and developing them. Pure happiness comes when a person does what he/she loves. When a person follows his/her passion, it is not work. It is a labor of love, and this is when the rewards are the highest. Children will excel when they pursue this as well. "Love what you do, and do what you love." This is life at its best.

Many people are amazed by the long hours and strenuous work that are required to find and make the natural medicines. They ask, "Why would you do that?" The answer is simple. It is due to a love of Nature. Helping others to attain higher goals and good health is a way to seek the highest path. Thus, to teach that people all must love this planet and take good care of it is only good sense. This is our human home. To destroy the earth—our home—its inhabitants and its resources with nuclear fallout, genetically engineered monstrosities, pesticides/herbicides, toxic wastes as well as garbage by the mountain load, and other noxious chemicals—is clearly insane. What the few in power do to the many has a lasting impact. Yet, power truly belongs to the many if the many will work together to make life better. That means educating people on the consequences of following the destructive trends versus seeking the rewards of building a better life, one step at a time. "The green revolution" is the common buzz all over the world. To help the world be a better place in every way can only make human life dramatically better.

Good parents must always be teachers. Yet, what is a good teacher? It means constantly learning new and better ways to live and function and then teaching this to the children. This is so much better than holding on to old ways and never changing and growing, while imposing their outdated belief systems onto the children.

Change is mandatory. There are now over 6.6 billion people on this planet. If every person merely picked up a piece of trash every day and properly disposed of it, such as recycling it, would it make a big difference? Certainly. For instance, it could save countless trees, which are the main source for purifying the air and providing oxygen. If $1.00 per person was spent every day on good, organic, nourishing food instead of junk food, would it make an impact? Absolutely. That's over $6.6 billion dollars a day. Now, that is power. The message would be loud and clear to manufacturers that we the people want what makes us strong, healthy, and intelligent.

If everyone walks or rides a bicycle whenever possible to each destination, every person will be more physically fit. This will save money on gasoline. Also, global warming and continuous destruction will be reduced. Interestingly, in the United States the price of gasoline rose during the Bush administration from $1.22 per gallon when George W. Bush, Jr. first came into office to as high as $5.00 per gallon in some places. The impact on the family budget was so great that people began driving less and less. This decrease in driving caused enough pressure on profit-taking to drop the price of fuel dramatically. In addition, it must be remembered that the decrease in driving also helped reduce pollution. It is still mandatory that better and more efficient means of transportation is achieved.

Every time another person is helped by learning better ways to live and thrive and the consequences of heedless destruction are finally revealed as well as understood, this is a big leap forward on the right path. The negative impossibilities of it all cannot be the focus. Of course, every single person on the earth will not cooperate. However, every individual who learns to think constructively and purposefully, while making an effort to stop indifferent consumption and destruction of resources, can make a difference.

It cannot be allowed that people who have no interest in individual welfare manage the day-to-day existence of every person, because then life is merely existence. When people succumb to mindlessly doing what they are told to do, whether it is through mandates or mass advertisements, no one benefits—not even those who are the controllers. Free thought allows for creation, our God-given right. Even what may seem like small decisions, such as letting children walk to school if it is close enough or growing a garden, even if it must be in containers, will help youngsters to be more responsible. They can better understand how even a small contribution *makes a difference* for the whole planet and adds to personal growth as well. This is the power of one. Kids need care, and they need to learn to care about themselves and others. We all do. Change for the better can happen, but everyone must work together to make it so.

Chapter One
Why Kids Need Care

The birth and rearing of a child is the most wonderful experience a couple can share. However, so many people bring children into the world without considering the major responsibility that child-bearing and then appropriate child care really are. This book is designed to help make this process easier, since planning for a child should begin well before conception. All children, including the developing embryo, need care. It's a common statement that babies don't come with an instruction book, but this information will help fill the void for those who seek guidance and answers.

Let's consider what it means that *Kids Need Care*. Both the father's and the mother's health are important to provide a strong beginning for an infant. This means that both parents need to be aware of the healthiest possible lifestyle and be willing to utilize healthy practices in their daily lives. Ideally, this begins with the quality and quantity of food that is consumed. It also includes practicing a daily exercise program as well as using truly clean water for drinking, cooking, and bathing and deeply breathing fresh air. It also means avoiding chemical contamination from such things as food dyes, smoking, alcohol, pesticides/herbicides, household and other chemicals, drugs—legal and illegal—

vaccinations, and any other potentially destructive intoxication. Remember, what is done to the body is passed on to the child. Radiation, including the overuse of ultrasound, should also be avoided, since it has been proven to be damaging to human tissue, especially a developing fetus. Souvenir sonograms of the developing infant have been the "in thing" for some time. Although lucrative, this is an irresponsible action of the caregiver. All the healthy practices are common sense, good habits to develop and maintain for a better quality life. This will ensure that the health and well-being of every family member is the best it potentially can be. Pregnancy and birth can be a dangerous time for the mother-to-be and the infant, so, certainly, a future father must actively pursue healthy life habits which will help limit his contribution to birth defects and abnormalities. It is important to adhere to the healthy practices and avoid the unhealthy ones such as smoking and the consumption of alcohol as well as drugs. This lessens the possibility for stress, strain, and serious health problems or abnormalities for the baby and difficult, even heartbreaking challenges for the parents.

There are many more challenges today for the family than ever before. Frequently, both parents are employed, and it is difficult to come home from work and be nurturing parents. Young executives, truck drivers, traveling salespeople, shift workers, hospital staff, military personnel, and many others in all sorts of professions may require long or varied working hours. Thus, today the effort required to maintain a reasonable income for a home and family are monumental. A stay-at-home mom or dad may feel left out of the employed spouse's life. Criticism and anger from either partner causes nothing but trouble for any relationship. Building understanding and a family lifestyle plan can help everyone to be more organized, to have more time to share for family activities, and to develop the desire and ability in each and every person in the family to be productive, happy, worry-free, and most of all—loving.

Without a plan time can slip away, and nothing is accomplished. The divine One says, *"It is not the number of your days, but the content of them that matters."* These are wise words that would be beneficial for everyone to remember. A ship never sails from a port without a destination and a log book. An airplane never leaves the ground without a flight plan. A country—and even an entire planet—falters when its leaders fail to lead with a viable road map for the future. Yet, so many people go through life without a clue regarding what paths their lives are following. There is no rule that every person must believe the same way and do the same things. Most assuredly, each person and every family is unique. It takes time and patience to learn about yourself and your family's needs, but it is worth it to build a guideline for each member of the family to follow.

While stresses and challenges in life can never be eliminated, how people handle them makes the difference. In other words, those inevitable bad events can be experienced as life-enhancing lessons or as major worries which threaten health and happiness. How "crisis" is handled is truly a personal choice. A person can choose to feel bad or be positive. As well, building a road map for life helps to get a perspective on where the journey is headed and what will happen on the way there. Massive changes in life may be required to obtain what an individual is capable of achieving. If destructive family practices were common in the past, change those negative patterns and avoid repeating them. It is important to learn to grow and change both for personal development as well as for the children's sake. It is important to never overreact because of negative life experiences. Often, when life has been a severe struggle for a person as a child and, then, wealth and ease are achieved as an adult, this individual swears that his/her children will never have to suffer as he/she did. The children are then so pampered that they become hopelessly spoiled. This is not beneficial for anyone.

Today, stress is a major factor for everyone. Life is fast-paced and complex. People are overwhelmed by the number of choices, decisions, and actions that are required in every-day living. By developing a flexible lifestyle plan which is suitable for all the personalities within the family unit, much of the stress of family interaction is relieved. This is particularly true with diet and nutrition. In the family unit, especially, a solid routine is invaluable. Children need reliable and responsible parents. This greatly relieves their stress burden and helps them to become, ultimately, reliable and responsible adults. When life gets out of balance, and there is no strong support system in place, a stressful environment is created. The problem is life is sort of like the teeter-totter. There are ups and downs, and it takes effort to maintain a balance. Likewise, it takes constant effort and caring to maintain an enduring family relationship.

The current trend of asking the children for guidance and decisions which they are incapable of making has caused great stress and agitation among the young. It also gives them power and control, which they are not prepared to handle. For example, while walking through the city aquarium souvenir store in Hawaii, I overheard a woman in a loud voice discussing where she and a companion would go for dinner. Then, she asked what would be best to eat and what time should they go. There seemed to be no reply to her questions. As I walked around the counter display, I rather expected to see a lady talking on a cell phone to another adult. Instead, she was talking to a small boy around three years old who was busy tearing the place apart. Regardless, he was far too young to be making the decisions for both of them. When a child is old enough to concentrate and reason, designated available choices can be explained, and then, he/she can help select from those choices. That is a learning experience. Yet, the power position as the parent/ leader and final decision maker has not been relinquished.

Because every person in a family is unique and no two humans or families are exactly alike, there are no concrete answers for every situation except to be considerate of the needs and feelings of each family member. Furthermore, each person reacts differently to the same situation. For example, the Taylors (not their real names) are a family of four: Lizbeth—Mom, Jeffrey—Dad, Jamie—number one son, and Darren—number two son. On a Thursday night as they were preparing for bed the phone rang. The call was from Mr. Taylor's father and mother—Gordon and Gloria Taylor. They would be flying in for the weekend, and they would be arriving around 7:00 p.m. on Friday (tomorrow) and leaving at 4:00 p.m. on Sunday. Lizbeth was stunned. Jeffery was an only child, and his well-to-do parents lived a very elegant and organized life. As she glanced around the room she was ready to panic. The house was a mess, and dirty laundry was seemingly reproducing itself in the laundry room. She was scheduled to be a teacher's assistant tomorrow, and a healthy snack was yet to be made. There was no fresh food, clean sheets or towels, and simply no time to make it all happen.

Jeffrey was baffled by the call and last minute announcement of a visit from his father. His parents always planned everything months in advance. He was a bit concerned, because of the mysterious circumstances of the surprise visit. He even felt a little irritated, because he had a full schedule planned on Saturday with clients and an outing with the boys on Sunday. Still, Jeffrey was delighted to know that they would be seeing his parents so soon. It had been over a year since he had last seen them.

Being the first grandson Jamie was Gordon's favorite. Jamie was so excited to show his grandfather how much he had grown, how fast he could run, and how his basketball skills had improved. Also, Grandpa Gordon always brought cool presents and slipped him a stash of spending money. Yet, it was kind of sad that the Sunday hike with his dad and Darren would be cancelled. They had planned it for a month, and the three of them had so little time together.

Darren knew "Nanna Gloria" would have something special for him. She always remembered to bring him a big surprise. He loved her stories and her attentive ear for his questions and comments. No one else ever had time to listen to him. "Oh—the Sunday hike. Who cares. I didn't want to go anyway, and Nanna Gloria will love my personal web page I designed," Darren thought to himself.

Gordon and Gloria knew that the short notice could cause some problems, so they made their plans convenient for everyone. They stayed in a lovely hotel, and all parties agreed that meals would be eaten there. Lizbeth was very relieved and, finally, was able to relax. They didn't even ask to come over to the house.

Jeffrey was so excited to show his parents his growing business, and he even introduced them to one of the scheduled clients. It turned out that the others were easily rescheduled. What at first appeared to be major challenges for Jeffrey were actually easily reconciled.

On Friday evening Jamie stayed with his grandparents at the hotel. After a beautiful meal and visit with the entire family, Gordon and Jamie headed for the workout room in the hotel. There, Jamie aptly demonstrated his physical prowess for his admiring grandfather. Of course, he couldn't wait to try out all the new games and other gifts that his grandparents brought.

Darren spent Saturday night with his grandparents at the hotel, and he and Nanna Gloria had a leisurely breakfast buffet on Sunday morning. He showed her his web page which she found to be fascinating, and as always, she was full of stories and surprises. Darren was so happy to be the center of attention and to actually be admired and rewarded for being the "geek" in the family.

Jeffrey, Gordon, and Jamie went for an early morning hike on Sunday, and they watched the sun rise together. This was a first, and they each experienced feelings that they didn't know existed. A rare bonding experience resulted between the three Taylor males.

Lizbeth even had a rare day to herself until they all went to the airport to send the happy twosome home. She needed some time to rest and organize her own thoughts and responsibilities. In the quiet and peace of the day she realized that anger and frustration were overwhelming her ability to cope. Changes were definitely needed, but she had been too busy to even realize they were necessary.

Why did the elder Taylors surprise the young family? Gordon's best friend died suddenly, and his own mortality loomed in his mind along with the pain of loss and sorrow.

During such times family ties become more important than ever—love *is* the answer. Emotionally, each of the younger Taylors reacted differently to the news of the visit according to their own personal interests. Emotions play a major role in how people act, what they say, and what they achieve in what seems important at the time. Yet, when love and consideration reign, all ends well.

What is the moral of this story? Family members can end up happy and fulfilled when everyone cooperates and considers the feelings of each other. In every situation consideration and caring are key factors. No one should carry the entire load in the family. No one individual is the slave or the servant, and the only Lord and Master is our creator. Ideally, everyone works together, including the children. All children, boys included, need to learn to be independent, self-sufficient, and, thus, self-confident with the daily tasks of life.

Some parents think they are honoring their children by giving them everything they could possibly want. They believe that to make children clean up after themselves, to learn to cook—even just simple things, to look after their clothes and personal belongings, and to perform household chores are merely forced actions that rob them of their childhood. This is a dire mistake. There are seriously rich people that cannot function, cannot so much as make a cup of instant soup without help. This is creating helplessness and cheating children out of learning necessary life skills. Plus, needless aggravation is inflicted on the caregiver, if children are not required to have family and household responsibilities. No doubt, it does take time to teach them. Additionally, they may never do the tasks with great proficiency. However, patiently and lovingly working with them and recognizing a job well done gives them confidence and skills upon which to build. Parents must especially agree to support each other in the practice of discipline, even if it requires counseling to establish a consistent and agreeable routine. When children detect dissention in the ranks, discipline is challenged. Then, chaos is inevitable. This is apparently a major problem today, because some of the most popular television shows are about child-rearing. English nannies first observe and then help families turn little terrors into little lambs. However, remember in every case the parents have to reform too. Children learn from those around them. The "Do as I say, not do as I do" philosophy is catastrophic. The "My children are always right. They can do no wrong" or "I love them too much to discipline them" philosophies are also destructive to children. This interferes with their personal development and creates an unhappy home. Remember, it takes work to make anything worthwhile and special, but anything special is worth the effort. Parents who expect their children to merely follow their example without any verbal guidance— without open communication—are in for a major disappointment. Why? How do you know what their interpretations and perceptions of your actions really are? Kids need loving care, and they need parental counsel. They also need thoughtful, *consistent* discipline. Their problems and questions may seem like little silly stuff, but parental input creates the foundation for the rest of their lives.

Some parents may not have had much guidance as children. Others may have been abused or were raised in a dysfunctional atmosphere. All of these parents, no doubt, need guidance. The solution may be self-imposed research and reading. Guidance from experts, such as the English nannies, who have helped so many, may prove invaluable. Yet, like so many families on the television shows, the old habits frequently resume as soon as the nanny leaves or the books are put back on the shelves. It requires personal responsibility to take action and make the appropriate choices to learn and grow mentally, emotionally, and spiritually. At best this includes both parents working together. However, at the least they must not work against each other in a continuous battle for control of the hearts and minds of the children. This also applies to parents who are divorced. Remember that there was once enough love to bring the child/children into this world. The child/children is/are the creation(s) of both parents. The point is to always seek the best for the child/children and to focus on the highest good. They are not pawns to be used to punish or manipulate the ex-spouse. What is done or left undone will have an impact on the child/children both spiritually and emotionally for the rest of their lives.

There is a vast amount of research and information about what affects a person's personality. Every human being is different, not to mention that every other living creature on the earth is also unique. This alone is a miracle. Regarding this uniqueness there are books on birth order and personality in relation to facial features, body shape, and size. There are also books on the role of gender, spiritual, and moral influences, nurture versus nature as well as the power of attitude in molding a person. Most parents are concerned about physical growth and well-being, but it is the spiritual growth that is the true reason for our existence. It is vital that everyone seeks to continue to improve the intellect and understanding and develop as much wisdom as possible throughout the duration of a lifetime on this earth.

Incorporating the golden rule into everything that is done is the ultimate achievement—by serving others as one wishes to be served. Children learn by imitation. It is especially important that the child or children see Mom and Dad interacting with others in respectful, caring, kind, friendly, thoughtful, understanding ways. In other words, parents are teaching their young, while they are acting as they desire others to likewise perform. Then, emotionally and physically healthy youngsters are inclined to do the same. This is especially true if their observations are reinforced by the parents explaining to them that this is a wonderful and appropriate way to live. Love and the golden rule are so important that no other human behavior can compare.

As mentioned previously many factors play a major role in the way the child acts and responds and the development of that individual. Are there any other messages you can derive from the Taylor family? Absolutely, there are. Birth order, for example, plays a significant role in the way people act throughout their lives. The birth order of Jeffrey's parents is unknown, but the fact that Jeffrey is an only child is known. The only child is accustomed to being acknowledged. He/she is the center of attention throughout childhood. This is great during the good times but not so great during the bad. While the only child is generally doted upon and receives more attention and material goods during childhood than others, he/she is also held responsible for his/her actions. This is merely because there are no other children around to spread the blame. The single child in a family is sometimes called the "lonely only," since there is no companionship with other siblings. Likewise, the only child does not experience the fighting and squabbling among siblings, so he/she doesn't learn negotiating skills as early. The only child has trouble doing things alone, even as an adult. For example, when asked to hang a picture, this particular person will need someone to find the nails, the hammer, and a ladder. Then, someone must mark the wall, put the hanger or wire on the back of the picture, and hold the nail and the ladder. Only then he/she will hammer in the nail. Even if this is quite an exaggeration, the minimum he/she will require is for someone to watch what he/she is doing and then require whatever help is perceived as needed. The point is this individual needs to be noticed and desires to be praised. When he/she doesn't get this attention, there may be payback with dirty tricks or emotional outbursts or even withdrawal. Jeffrey needed his parents' approval and was delighted that they could see his burgeoning business. Between fathers and sons there is frequently a certain amount of competition. Jeffrey's father, being highly successful, was an extra challenge for him, and he really needed his father's blessings. This is especially so, since Mr. Taylor had been critical of Jeffrey in the past.

Lizbeth, Jeffrey's wife, was a middle child, and this is always a good match for oldest or only children, who are always more demanding and like to maintain control. Middle children are generally the pacifists depending on where they fall in the family lineup. As children they do not have the power base, the freedoms, or the responsibilities of the oldest child. Nor do they have the last "chick in the nest" allowances that the youngest always gets. They are either too young to do what the eldest does or too old to do what the youngest does. They usually try to negotiate peace, and they do whatever it takes to do so. Lizbeth was a pleaser, so she tried to do it all. In trying to please everyone, she failed even to please herself. Lizbeth didn't even know she had the right to feel overwhelmed. Also, she was frequently angry and frustrated, when her "three boys" dumped everything on her. Jeffrey, being an only male child from a wealthy family, was no help in the household and had no manual skills whatsoever. Although successful his business was still developing, so household help was not yet feasible. Therefore, he left everything about the home to her. Yet, she was responsible for their inconsiderate actions. Being a middle child, it was difficult for her to establish household rules for the family. Thus, they expected her to be the family slave. This was not only unfair to Lizbeth, but it was unfair to the other family members as well. The males in the family were totally helpless in accomplishing mere simple tasks such as fixing even a quick meal or a snack, washing a load of clothes without destroying them, and maintaining an orderly environment. Frequently, the slave or victim personality is fearful of training and guiding others to be self-sufficient. This is because such action also relinquishes a certain amount of personal control and the dependency of others. The time by herself gave her an opportunity to reflect on her own life and emotions. However, she realized that she needed help to sort out all the feelings and then to start building a better understanding of herself and her family.

Jamie, the firstborn son, was a new and exciting experience for his parents and grandparents. From the beginning they couldn't take their eyes off of this new heir, and they noticed every smile and responded to his every cry. Here, it is important to note that even babies learn quickly how to control and manipulate their environment if parents aren't aware and prepared with loving discipline. That means disciplining themselves as well in order not to spoil the child. You may think absolutely everything the child does is cute and brilliant, but it is guaranteed that others will not. It is only fair that a child should be aware of socially acceptable behavior and his/her place in the world. Otherwise, the child will carry inappropriate behavior into adulthood and will suffer the consequences. One young man who was always allowed to do as he pleased as a child now claims, "If I didn't have bad luck, I wouldn't have any luck at all." It is virtually impossible to convince him that he is responsible for the consequences of his own inappropriate actions.

Usually, oldest children are said to be the most successful, but this is not an absolute rule. All children in the family realm have hidden talents, which are like blossoms waiting to open. Some children cope or even thrive on their own, and others always need more encouragement. The oldest child, like Jamie, desires the approval of his/her elders. Grandfathers and grandsons usually relate even better than fathers and sons. However, control is the issue here. It is the human pecking order, and the oldest of every generation wants the power. This will play out throughout the rest of their lives. That is why the oldest will need a middle child or a baby of the family as a spouse. Two oldest children together spell certain disaster, because there will always be a battle for control and acknowledgement. This is true unless they are aware of these birth order idiosyncrasies and continuously work to make allowances for them in their relationship.

Generally, the oldest are accustomed to responsibility, and they either work hard or are directing others. However, watch out for retaliation, when they don't get their way or if they can't have the controlling influence at work or play. Most won't even recognize these traits in themselves and will be angry if this is mentioned to them. Most will heartily deny that such nonsense could be true. Introspection and self analysis are so necessary for everyone, because it is always most difficult to know and understand oneself.

Now, it is important to recognize the role son number two plays in the Taylor family. A second son will nearly always be the total opposite of the first born. If the first born is meticulous and responsible, the second born will be the opposite. If the first son is an athlete and is very stoical, the second son will be the geek and quite likely will be a whiner. In other words, if you know what son number one is like, son number two will be uniquely different. The oldest son will most likely taunt and tease the younger boy.

The following is a true example of two brothers, who were less than a year apart in age. The oldest boy and his friends made the younger boy absolutely miserable whenever possible. They warned the younger boy to keep his mouth shut, or he would be treated even worse. The younger boy was afraid to tell his parents of the maltreatment. However, son number one was quite meticulous and loved to make model planes. He would carefully work for hours until they were perfect. One day the older boy and his friends inflicted a particularly intense abusive harassment session upon the younger boy. While the younger boy was always the peacemaker, he finally had had enough. He took his brother's perfect model planes to the garage, poured glue all over them, and set them on fire. Since the garage almost caught fire too, the parents finally became aware that there was a problem.

While both boys are now successful men, the older son still tries to demean and defeat the younger. This behavior is extreme, especially since the younger man is far more important and prosperous in his chosen field than his jealous brother. For peace of mind and emotional survival the younger son must keep many miles between himself and his brother. The younger brother is learning to no longer be his brother's or anyone else's victim. Still, the older brother continues to resist growth and change. Even after long separations the older brother will inflict torment whenever there is an opportunity.

If the second child in the Taylor family had been a sister, a different reaction from number one son would have occurred. He would have been her protector. He might have still been somewhat abusive at times, but he most likely would be her defender and advocate for life. Yet, unfortunately, this birth order pattern can become an incestuous relationship, so do not let this happen for the welfare of both children. Never ignore signs of tension and fear between the two, even though this is not easy for a parent to even consider. When there is deep abiding pure love and caring in the family structure, it will not. Pure love is sincere, unconditional, and free of motive.

There are many books that reveal far more information about the various actions and reactions of people within a family unit. It is important to know and understand everything you possibly can. Family relations extend into every part of a person's life. Such knowledge can make another person's behavior almost predictable whether at work, at home, or at play.

Raising a family is the best of life experiences, and yet, it is the most difficult of life experiences. Every person must learn lessons, and people were put together for a reason. It is not an accident. Everything that happens in life is an opportunity to know and understand more, even when the lessons are bitter ones. When an open mind is maintained, the bad experiences can actually help individuals make better choices. It is important to make this life a positive experience. Like the young man who says he only has bad luck, whatever the mind's focus is, that is the result, good or bad. It is most difficult to recognize personal thoughts and actions that cause self defeat. It is always easier to see what the other fellow has done, right or wrong.

Personally, it is important to feel good about all things done well, and yet be forgiving of any mistakes. When a scene is shot for a film or movie, the director yells action and then calls it a "take," when it is finally good enough to use. Rarely is the first scene acceptable, and the final take may require dozens of repeated performances. So a mistake is merely an action that did not work out as desired—a "mis" take. In life it is called learning, when the next time that same action in some form is done correctly. Thus, it becomes a "take" instead of a mistake.

Building the family bond

Sharing time together is the best way of bonding for a lifetime. Jennifer, the oldest child in the Patterson family and a bit of a tomboy, loves to go to the big amusement parks and always chooses the wildest rides. Shannon, her younger sister, is a petite little lady and loves nothing wilder than the merry-go-round. Sean, the baby of the family, is all boy, and he likes to play the games and win the prizes.

The children are all young enough that adult supervision is still necessary. Without a prearranged agreement this family outing could turn into total chaos. Mom loves the wild rides too, so she and Jennifer plan their agenda. Dad agreed to stay with the two younger children, and they spilt the time equally between the gentler rides and the games. Dad had to help out with the games, because Sean needed assistance to win those prizes he wanted so much. Since Shannon is always so patient, she won the big pink fuzzy bunny award. At a designated time and place they all rejoined and had a lovely homemade picnic in the park. The kids already knew that the sugary junk food was off limits, and there were no complaints.

There are lots of clues and hidden information in this little family adventure. As mentioned earlier a simple plan for the day helped the little outing to be fun and enjoyable for all. When chaos reigns, no one knows what to expect or what to do next. Simple ground rules that are established early on make life easier for parents and children. However, parents' attitudes change as more children join the family. The older children tend to believe that the baby of the family gets by with "murder" compared to what they were allowed to do. Frequently, they develop an endless jealousy over this. Then, the baby of the family is jealous of the fact that the older children get to do so much more than he/she does. Again the middle child tends to be the peace maker/moderator of all the siblings. Birth order plays a huge role in how everyone acts and reacts to every situation in life. Learn it, know it, use it to understand everyone around, and make life more interesting and enjoyable.

The more understanding and clear the communication between parents and children, the easier it is to cope with day to day events. It's the little things that accumulate and cause the conflicts. Knowledge is bliss. Ignorance is not. When family guidelines are established from infancy, children know the boundaries and consequences. This is critical to maintain peace and happiness within the family unit. It is also necessary to help parents maintain their wisdom and their sanity. Children are always testing their limits. Yet, with rules and guidelines established with love, children feel secure and are less likely to be demanding and uncontrollable. Giving the power to them will create only nightmares and a multitude of unmanageable moments. Children look to parents for strength and guidance. They want to be led, not to lead. That is why it is important to establish the following three steps early on:

1. Write out a book of house rules, and make sure the children know them and understand them.

2. Always be consistent—don't change the rules around on a whim or be firm one time and slipshod another.

3. Let them know there are consequences to inappropriate behavior. Explain those consequences. Make it clear and easy to understand. Follow up with those consequences when necessary. This includes time out, the naughty stool or mat for the little ones, or curfews and loss of privileges and money for older children. Children don't need or want to be treated mean. When they are certain that you love them, but not their bad behavior, you have achieved a balance in the family unit. There are exceptions to rules, but any exception should be given careful deliberation, thoroughly discussed, and seldom allowed. Rules also change as children grow older and as their wants and needs increase and acceptance of responsibility develops.

Rage and anger are major disruptors within an individual. Fear is another, and actually, rage and anger are forms of fear. No matter which family member experiences these negative feelings, they are powerful emotions and must be dealt with immediately and thoroughly. The pain that these emotions bring into the lives of all involved is too great if left unchecked. Drinking, drugs, all types of addictions and inappropriate behavior will result if these negative emotions are not addressed. Family love or family trouble can be passed on from generation to generation. If you came from a troubled family, seek help now.

The following true story is an example of how misery is passed on through the generations. A very unhappy woman came from a deeply troubled family. She was worked like a farm animal and beaten frequently. Thus, she continued doing what she knew best. Her form of discipline included screaming, beating, berating, and demeaning. Yet, among all the crude, violent discipline that she inflicted, there was only one thing her daughter remembered actually doing wrong. Ironically, it was her words that modified her daughter's behavior for the better—not the beatings.

When the girl was around seven years old, she ate some junk food in the living room. Upon finishing the snack, she wiped her hands on the arm of the couch. The mother merely said in a calm and low voice, "Some day you will have a home of your own, and you won't like it when people wipe their dirty hands on your furniture." The girl never forgot that one instance, and, yet, she could not tell you what precipitated all the beatings and screaming fits.

What is the lesson? Make the punishment fit the "crime." Try to stay calm, and never lash out in anger. Make sure the child understands what behaviors are unacceptable and why. Most importantly, make sure that the child knows you love him/her but not what he/she is doing. It is also necessary that it is clearly understood that you mean business.

Oprah Winfrey expressed her admiration for her friend Gayle who established that she was the parent in charge early on with her family. Her daughter spouted off one day, and Gayle said, "Who do you think you are talking to like that?" The little one looked down and sheepishly said, "my shoes." Mom was definitely in charge, but what a fast thinking creative answer. Children can be so funny, but it is important to maintain composure as well as a sense of humor. They need to know you are serious about correcting behavioral actions before those actions become problems.

Do not succumb to a battle of arguments. It is tough to stand firm. It is much easier to give in, but ultimately all parties will be thankful for maintaining a just and firm stand. Just think of it as another lesson for everyone. Time passes so fast, and children grow up so quickly. It is critical that they are prepared for life's lessons as best as possible.

Children are the treasures of God, but there will be some days and nights that this tender thought may seem doubtful. Remember that life is a continuous learning experience for all family members. Unfortunately, there are many families that have significant difficulties. Moreover, many may not even be aware that there are problems. Some are aware of their problems but are unable to solve them. It is very difficult to find the answers and make the changes that are so critical, when emotional/spiritual problems are deeply rooted. This is especially so, if there is no apparent help. Our great creator is always ready to comfort and lift up hearts and souls, when they are offered in prayer or meditation. Truly, no one is ever alone, and this only needs to be accepted with the firmest of faith. Such blessings are readily available for the asking. Remember to pray/meditate and ask for guidance. This is a time of learning for everyone. Be patient, forgiving, caring, fair, and, most of all, loving. When gratitude fills the heart, negativity will never overpower the joy from within. Nothing can overwhelm the blessings from the light.

There are no perfect mortal beings, so "mis-takes" will be made. Forgiveness and laughter are two important healing ingredients. Being able to readily forgive and laugh at personal foibles and mistakes makes life easier. The most important point is to know that the best efforts have been made according to the abilities and skills that are available. However, remember that with a little effort, better ways to accomplish most anything can usually be found. Also, the most important habit is "do not worry." Save that huge amount of energy that worry requires for productive, positive thinking. Keep the peace within. Know that the eternal spirit is learning and growing. Life is what each person decides it will be. Life *is* what a person *thinks*.

Finally, keep in mind that it is the parent who gets to be in charge. If a child is allowed to constantly eat any kind of junk, watch endless hours of television or play computer games, and be totally sedentary and unproductive, a futile pattern is set. Parents are astonished and wonder what went wrong when this child acts out, and indulges in alcohol, drugs, and other misadventures. They consider themselves good and caring parents, who have provided everything the child ever wanted. Yet, this child has not learned to focus and be disciplined in thought and deed. Sometimes the poor parents are working endlessly to provide a better life for their children so that the children do not have any hardships. Yet, those hardships were the necessary fire that tempered the steel of their own personal resolve and strength of character.

Sometimes what seems like a nightmare will cause a person to become an extraordinary being. There is a young lady who has lived and worked through a debilitating experience. She has fought to survive, and she is extraordinary. As a youngster because of her illness she must consistently eat and drink only that which is nourishing. She regularly takes nutritional supplements as well as exercises daily. This has tremendously increased her performance. Her focus is so consistent that she is voted the best student year after year. This delicate little flower has already achieved more than many adults. In spite of the hardship she has learned to focus, to grow and develop, and to use her skills productively at a very young age.

Many people think that children should not be pressed to do anything but play and have so-called fun and a good time. Anything otherwise they consider tyranny for their children. However, there are consequences. These same children need to be entertained continuously. They are constantly bored. They want a good time and somebody to provide it. Meanwhile, this delicate little lady knew at an early age how fleeting life is, and she is using her time on this planet in hugely productive ways.

What do you think the pampered, good-time Charlie type does for himself or anyone else? He does nothing, because he is looking for others to dote over him. He'll yammer for donuts and sodas, while his body is faltering under the sugar-chemical load. Then he'll expect everyone to drop everything and run to the hospital to console him with chocolates, flowers, and lots of pity while the doctors test and prod to try to find some physical abnormality/disease to explain his many adverse symptoms. Some people never find the answers, the peace, the love that they so sorely need.

Children require discipline and guidance. Discipline doesn't mean beatings and screaming at the top of the lungs and ordering them around every minute of their lives. It means establishing set rules and fundamental guidelines, which begin at infancy. There will be changes as the child matures and is able to accept more responsibility. This system includes established times to sleep and to awaken, a family eating schedule, responsibilities for the care of self, awareness of the rights of each family member, and respect for the home. This planet operates according to a clock. There are set times for most activities such as work, school, vacations, and holidays. The happy and healthy child has an easier time functioning within the flow of life patterns.

The most successful and happy people have enough energy to fulfill all that they need to accomplish, and they do it in some kind of a formatted way. Fun, laughter, and joy must be a part of life, but they must also be part of the growth process of the mind, heart, and soul. A mindless shoveling down of addictive commercial junk not even fit to be called food does not nourish the body. The feeding of the brain of the same type of mindless drivel that is commonly accepted as entertainment does not increase the intellect. Finally, the total lack of focus on the enlightenment that makes the spirit soar will not help any person reach his or her highest potential. Just as it takes work to make a garden grow and provide beautiful produce, children must be guided and directed and taught with love. In addition, the child must be allowed to use his/her creative genius and be the person that the soul reveals. Then, this child will be the amazing being he/she is meant to be.

In their thoughts and actions children are free spirits. Typically, parents undermine this free nature with endless restrictions, control, and demands. With all this loss of personal freedom the results are a stifling of creativity and curiosity, which is a loss beyond comprehension. There must be guidance and discipline, but every child must be allowed to strive in his/her own way and, thus, thrive as an individual.

Every action has its consequences. This can be beneficial or harmful. Be honorable and good towards children, and it will create more of the same. In contrast, just as decency and human kindness elevate society, greed and unlimited power ultimately bring its destruction.

Every child is unique. One child may be more compatible with the parent(s) than another. However, this does not mean that something is wrong with the child who is not favored. He/she is just different. Everyone has talents, abilities, and excellence of some kind. Look for it, and help each child to develop his/her own individual magic.

Chapter Two

Food for Babies

When we arrive here on the earth, the first nourishment we get is air, and that is when life begins. Air is the most important life-giving agent, and oxygen is the nutrient that makes the blood red. Every cell is a tiny living life force, and all cells must have oxygen to grow (divide) and function. Each cell has mitochondria, which function as its lungs. This special combination of billions of cells makes up a new human life force that requires clean air to survive and thrive. That's why everyone anxiously awaits that first breath of life from the newly born baby.

The next nourishment is ideally from the mother. Breast milk is the naturally correct food for a baby, and it helps to establish and strengthen the immune system for the duration of the individual's life. So, thank you, mothers, for your enduring contribution. Every nutrient needed in the right proportion should be available to make the child grow and thrive. Of course, if the mother's diet is poor, the milk will be affected, and both mother and child will suffer the negative consequences and ill health of malnutrition.

Sometimes, nursing is not an option. Either the baby or the mother or both are not physically able to proceed. Still, optimum nutrition during pregnancy should prevent this from happening. Mother's milk is the perfect food. Also, nursing is the time for bonding between mother and child.

It was quite the fad for awhile that babies were bottle fed. It made life less restrictive for Mom, so it caught on fast. Mothers were led to believe that formula was equally as good as breast milk or even better. Except in the direst cases of nutritional deficiency or illness, this is absolutely false. Also, most formulas are made from cow's milk or soybeans. Both are suspect now. Cow's milk may be suspect because of the way the animals are fed, drugged, and vaccinated. Soy is suspect because it is genetically engineered. During pollination it is further exposed to GMO material. The soybean also contains compounds which make it difficult to digest and may be toxic in a brand new body with an undeveloped digestive system. Neither cow's milk nor soy supplies the correct balance of nutrients. Furthermore, other commercial formulas contain too much synthetic material for such a delicate little system to be safely nourished.

Pasteurized cow's milk is known for causing infant gastritis and colic. Plus, in the United States it is likely to be contaminated with bovine growth hormone. It may even be infected with encysted parasites from rendered animal by-products, which are fed to the cows. Parasites, and especially the cysts, may survive pasteurization.

Cows are not carnivores and should never be fed animal parts, yet, they are. In cows this dangerous practice has led to "mad cow" disease. Thus, Creutzfeld Jacob disease may develop in humans who consume contaminated products. Dr. Cass Ingram, renowned nutritional physician, author, and media expert, says that this practice could potentially lead to "mad milk." Then, he notes, this will jeopardize the infant's health and development. If a cow's milk formula is considered, only organic milk should be used. Yet, it should also be remembered that any form of cow's milk is not the ideal food for infants. Therefore, at the first sign of gastrointestinal upset and vomiting, change to a different milk source from goats or sheep or, even better, human milk. Raw milk from women who have been tested for diseases such as AIDS is available.

While "mad milk" is a relatively new concern, bovine growth hormone is a more commonly recognized danger. It causes infection (mastitis) in the udders of cows, and the milk is contaminated with pus. Plus, the hormone remains in the milk and affects the growth and weight of the child. Researchers have found evidence that growth hormone can even cause cancer. It has been reported that young teenage girls who have consumed large quantities of milk each day have developed breast cancer. Cast your vote for better milk and all other food with your buying power by purchasing organic and raw whenever possible.

A formula that is still recommended and used by many new mothers is a combination of canned milk and corn syrup. There are three major problems with this concoction. First, the canned milk is not organic. Secondly, the milk is cooked at a high degree of temperature, and it is hardly digestible for an adult let alone an infant digestive system. Thirdly, the corn syrup is, no doubt, made from genetically engineered corn, which is causing severe allergic reactions. Furthermore, it is harmful to the undeveloped pancreas as are all processed sugars. This is not proper nourishment for a baby. This was a common formula used in the 1950s, and many of those who still survive such a beginning are obese. Many others suffer from alcohol addiction and cardiovascular problems and are steadily developing adult onset diabetes and other health problems and complaints. Asthma and breathing difficulties are also common as well as skin rashes and candida yeast infections.

Other common infant formulas also cause difficulties. For example, there are several major problems with soy milk. Around 80% of soybeans are from genetically engineered sources, and even the organic soybeans are suffering the consequences of cross-pollination. Therefore, total contamination of all soy in the United States is only a matter of time. No research has been done to determine the full extent of the consequences of the alteration of such a major food source. However, when bacterial and viral components are injected into the genetic matter of a plant, there is no guarantee what will happen next. Undoubtedly, allergic reactions are certain to occur, and that is just the beginning of bizarre health issues, genetic damage, and, perhaps, even sudden unexplained deaths.

A scientific study sponsored by the FDA was done in France using a genetically engineered drug. The children involved in the testing had weak immune systems. The drug was supposed to revive their immune systems, and yet, three of the children died. As a result the study was cancelled. This certainly demonstrates that there is a definite danger with the irresponsible and monopolistic genetic engineering methods.

Further proof occurred when a Japanese company manufactured a genetically engineered tryptophan, which caused an allergic immune response called eosinophillia. Over fifty people died. All tryptophan was seized and removed from pharmacies and health food stores—even the types that were not genetically engineered. However, tryptophan is still added to infant formula, since it is an essential amino acid needed for growth and development. Yet, no one knows if it is genetically engineered or not. It most likely is. If it is, no one knows the long range health consequences of this untested and untried material. Due to massive lobbying and exchange of substantial sums of money, the companies responsible for this aberration of nature are never forced to prove the safety of such experimental foods and drugs.

While strict labeling requirements are enforced on food supplements in health stores and the internet with millions of dollars of fines for merely mentioning a potential cure or treatment, absolutely nothing is required—not even labeling—for these potentially deadly altered foods, which unsuspecting people consume daily. Ultimately, it will be too late to require labeling, when all food will be damaged by the cross pollination, which inevitably occurs. This should be considered as a cause for unexplained sudden infant death syndrome and other fatalities in children. To obtain important information for the protection of the family welfare refer to OrganicConsumers.com. At this time the only way to combat such tyranny is to refuse to buy any genetically engineered products or drugs. The aforementioned website will help to make that determination. The government has denied all citizens the right to make an educated choice by refusing to mandate that these freak GMO-contaminated foods and drugs must be labeled. Yet, labeling requirements for natural nutritional supplements are more draconian every year.

To continue there are further difficulties with soy that exist as well. The orientals have used soy as a staple in their diets for centuries but only in the fermented forms such as soy sauce, miso, and tempe. Tofu is a soy curd, so it is not fermented. Since soy is a legume, it is difficult to digest, even for adults. The Japanese would never dream of drinking soy milk, let alone doing so on a daily basis. Babies are fragile creatures, and their tiny systems are just beginning to adapt to life on earth. Soy contains highly indigestible substances called lectins, which may cause allergy and intestinal toxicity. It also contains a high amount of copper. This mineral antagonizes the absorption of zinc. It is zinc which is important for the breakdown and utilization of protein. It is also needed for growth and repair of tissue. In addition, zinc is necessary for enzyme production in digestion and the elimination of carbon dioxide. When a soy-based formula is used exclusively, the infant will almost certainly develop problems, particularly digestive and also respiratory.

There is yet another serious danger. This is because soy contains a high amount of estrogenic compounds. Some male children have developed female-like breasts on a high soy diet. Girls are also maturing earlier than ever before. The estrogenic compounds are taken up by the estrogen receptor cells, and thus, the absorption of natural estrogen is blocked. Needless to say, the consequences are potentially disastrous and may lead to cancer.

In infants and children soy is also a major cause of allergy and asthma. It may also play a role in the outbreak of eczema. A steady diet of soy foods and snacks, such as soy milk, chips, burgers, dogs, nuts, ice cream, cheese, shakes, oil, protein, and bars, is not recommended for any family member. This, of course, especially includes pregnant or nursing mothers. However, the organic fermented soy foods can be enjoyed occasionally, if there is no allergic reaction.

Soy formula should be avoided unless there is no other option and then only if it is derived from an organic source. Soy is dangerously low in thiamine and riboflavin as well as calcium and iodine. In contrast whole milk is generally rich in such nutrients. While soy is a fairly good source of essential amino acids, methionine and cystine are deficient. Also, the growth of friendly bacteria such as lactobacillus, acidophilus, and bifidus, which support and aid digestion, are inhibited by the lack of milk sugar. Even though commercial ready-made formulas are fortified with some of the important missing nutrients, it is most certainly from synthetic additives, many of which are genetically engineered. Natural sources of nutrients are far more nourishing and readily absorbed by the baby's growing body than synthetic ones.

For infants who must be bottle-fed, there are not many suitable choices. One choice is goat's milk. However, it is lacking in certain nutrients, which must be added. It is low in vitamin A, folic acid, and vitamin C. Also, maternal milk is high fat and low carbohydrate in composition. It is ideal to try and match mother's milk as much as possible.

Many times babies appear limp, scrawny, and grayish-colored from being fed synthetic formulas. They have little or no vitality. Often, they suffer from digestive disturbances such as colic and constipation. Many are also afflicted with fungal infections and eczema. Changing the formula makes a huge difference, and there are pronounced improvements in a short time. Interestingly, the babies fed a fortified raw goat milk formula even have tone and muscle definition that is rarely seen today among the poorly fed population. Even so, mother's milk is always the most desirable, but lactation requires a mother to stay away from highly processed junk food, sugar, chocolate, and food dyes. It also requires that she avoid vegetables and meats contaminated with pesticides, herbicides, GMOs, and chemicals. The nursing mother should enjoy a wide variety of fresh, nourishing, organic food. This is important for the physical and mental health, as well as strength, of both mother and child. If the mother is improperly nourished, the child is as well. Babies suffer the consequences of poor quality breast milk with symptoms such as failure to thrive and grow. They may even contract nutritional diseases such as beri-beri. Nutritional deficiencies are common. Too many women have no idea how important a balanced diet of clean, healthy food is for both mother and child. Even though there is such a wealth of food in this country, the overall quality is poor. This is for a multitude of reasons. Poor quality, mineral deficient soil is one issue. Plus, synthetic fertilizers and other highly toxic chemicals are commonly used in farming. Genetically engineered seeds and heavy refining of processed foods contribute to the nutritional nightmare. Then, there is contamination of the air and water. Since the whole planet is contaminated, this affects every man, woman, and child. If it continues undaunted, the human race may not survive.

Scientists recently tested breast milk from women consistently eating the Standard American Diet. It was found to contain exceedingly high levels of pesticides, herbicides, mercury, and other chemicals. Women are constantly exposed to a multitude of household chemicals, pesticides and herbicides, fire retardants, formaldehyde, and more. Toxins are readily found in the blood and, therefore, breast milk as well. It seems this is an excretory means for ridding the body of such poisons. Some breast milk has been found to be more toxic than the placental blood. All mothers should attempt to cleanse their bodies of at least some of these toxins before conception. It is wise to avoid as many forms of contamination as possible. Bug sprays, oven cleaners, even clothing finishes can poison the system. Yet, there are foods and herbal concentrates that will purge the poisons. It takes effort to eat wisely and well. Fortunately, even commercial grocery stores are beginning to bend to the demands of people who are learning how important nutrition and clean organic or wild food is for the family.

Now, another dangerous substance is threatening our existence. The depleted uranium used in weaponry and bombs is being swept by the wind from war-torn countries, including those that the United States occupies. This is taking its toll in the country of its origin and manufacture. Doctors in Florida are reporting an increase in lung cancer due to the radioactive material in the winds. As always, infants and the elderly are affected first. In Iraq radiation exposure has caused countless horrible birth defects. This is because of the direct damage of the egg, sperm, and developing fetus. On the internet there are many pictures of the pitiful infants, who are so deformed that they do not appear to be human. For further information, pictures, and a detailed book refer to Dr. M. Miraki's website, www.afghanistanafterdemocracy.com. Likewise, many U.S. soldiers have constant exposure. The radioactive material is in their sperm or ovum virtually forever. Upon their husbands' return many military wives complain of vaginal burning from the semen. This radiation contamination is also adversely affecting any resultant babies.

The people of the world do not need a poisoned environment and nuclear war. Moreover, the human race cannot survive continuous exposure to noxious chemicals and radiation. These substances make this world more and more toxic, and the consequences are extremely severe, if not deadly, in every realm.

Science has proven repeatedly that good nutrition is the key to vitality, strength, energy, and a happy disposition.

Feeding the baby correctly with the nutrients it needs is especially important. Infancy is the most active growth period of the entire lifespan. This is the essential time period for establishing the foundation of health for this little person for the rest of its life. Every system of the body is affected. The cardiovascular system must be strong, because this determines the function of the heart, circulation, and cholesterol levels. The brain development determines the abilities of the individual. This affects the ability to learn and function physically, as well as mentally. While intelligence level is important, balanced mental stability is necessary to relate and communicate with others throughout life.

The creation of a strong immune system is the ideal protection from asthma, colds, flu, and many communicable diseases. Plus, with sound nutrition cancer, arthritis, diabetes, and other crippling killers are less likely to be a problem. To challenge the digestive system at this age with nutritionally poor food could result in allergies and intestinal disorders. It could also result in brain function disorders, epilepsy, fungal outbreak, and failure to thrive. The baby's skin should be soft and silky and have a fresh smell. Yet, many times the skin is the first place babies show a reaction. Even nursing mothers need to observe and take note of adverse reactions in infants after feedings. Mothers may need to change their diets accordingly.

For mothers who nurse there are two books which explain good eating habits. The first is *How to Eat Right and Live Longer* and the other is *Supermarket Remedies*, both by Dr. Cass Ingram. He explains what to eat, what not to eat, and how food is effective for maintaining good health. Eating right is critical during lactation. Nursing is even more nutritionally depleting for mothers than pregnancy.

For infants who must be bottle-fed, a nutrition professional should be consulted to recommend a natural formula. Don't worry about taste. Just because you don't like it doesn't mean the baby won't. However, if the baby consistently refuses to drink a formula, the cause may be due to intolerance to one or more of the ingredients. If a milk formula is used, find a source of organic goat or sheep milk. Raw milk is best, but it needs to be fortified with a drop or two of the best wild oregano oil per quart of milk. Mix well. Then, each day add a nutrient-rich ingredient such as Polar fish oil. If a reaction occurs with any addition, leave out that ingredient. When all symptoms cease, begin adding in any remaining natural (not synthetic) nutrients one at a time. Again, stop if any reaction occurs, since the baby may be sensitive to more than one ingredient. Every baby reacts differently. Therefore, symptoms of intolerance may include rash, colic/gas, sneezing, vomiting, continual fussiness, ear-ache (older babies pull on the ear), loose stools, or constipation. Animal milk of some form is always the most nourishing basic food for the infant. Yet, any milk will need fortification to even somewhat simulate human milk.

Human milk is raw milk. That means it is unpasteurized and still contains the raw enzymes, amino acids, and many other nutrients that are unaltered by heat. Therefore, all the nutrients for growth and development are available in the proper combination and balance for the immune system and physical dynamics of a healthy baby. Of course, if the mother is malnourished, the milk will not provide any missing substances unless they are derived from her own tissues. That is why it is so important for pregnant and nursing women to make every bite of food count for their own physical benefit as well as the baby's. Remember, that mother's milk is one of the most precious gifts that can be given to a baby in spite of what even some doctors or health professionals may claim.

Much of nutrition research begins in the animal world. Farm animals are a valuable resource, so a lot of research focuses on the best food for them. Therefore, they and other animals provide lessons for human nutrition as well. For example, there is a large wild cat rescue center in Colorado. The owners learned a valuable lesson when two abused large black leopards were rescued. The female surprised them with a tiny baby shortly after their arrival. The big cats were so frightened that they stayed hidden inside a small red cage. The people knew the cub would not survive, because the males usually kill the cubs. Also, the mother did not try to nurse the precious little black ball of fluff. They named the little fellow Eddie. He readily ate the cow's milk every four hours, but his growth was slow and his beautiful black fur came out in patches. Eddie tried to play, but he was so weak he could barely move. They decided to try different formulas, because it was apparent that Eddie would not live much longer. Finally, they developed a formula of dried puppy milk and water with raw eggs. Eddie loved it. He began to thrive and grow. His fur grew back, and his coat was beautiful. He was active and playful. Eddie is now a full grown, healthy leopard, but he would not have survived if his formula had not been changed. Human babies thrive and grow the best with human milk. They are stronger and healthier. Their immune systems are more powerful, so they usually are well, while other children seem to catch every infection.

Raw milk is always more nourishing than pasteurized and much easier to digest. Yet, now it is difficult if not impossible to buy raw milk of any kind. Pasteurization kills the friendly bacteria, destroys the raw enzymes, and causes the amino acids to be barely digestible. Milk can be contaminated with many germs, including the tuberculosis bacillus. Therefore, all raw milk must be derived from clean sources. A drop or two of wild oregano natural spice oil (handpicked Mediterranean source) in a quart of milk may lengthen the shelf life of the raw milk.

Laws for industrial standards do not necessarily coincide with the best interests of the human race. They are usually designed to cover up the dangers of inferior products. If animals were fed their healthy natural forage and good farming practices were observed, raw milk would not be a problem. However, currently the only alternatives you have for raw milk at this time is to breast-feed your baby, raise goats or sheep, or somehow find a source of raw milk—perhaps a wet nurse as they did in the olden times.

It cannot be overemphasized how important it is to feed a child its natural food. New mothers must mentally and physically prepare for breast-feeding before the baby is born. La Leche League in every community is a huge help. One of the founders stated she had difficulty with breast-feeding. However, she was determined to make it work and did just that. Then, she decided to help other young mothers. This group has been assisting young mothers with breast feeding for over 40 years. She noted that very few are unable to feed their babies, if they are determined to do so.

If it seems there is not enough milk for the child or that this type of feeding is inconvenient, there are solutions. Women adopting newborns are using various foods, herbs, and spices to induce milk production. Yes, they have never been pregnant, and they are breast-feeding their babies.

There are foods, herbs, and spices that will encourage a free flow of milk. Fenugreek and black seed seem to be helpful for many. There is also a mother's tea that has been beneficial for increasing milk production.

If you are working or must leave the infant for periods of time, express the milk with a pump and put it in a bottle. The milk can even be frozen, but this affects the enzymes and fresh is always better. Your baby will thank you for your efforts, when he/she grows up to be a strong and healthy adult.

Remember it was not long ago that wet nurses as they were called were hired to feed babies of the wealthy or for babies whose mothers could not produce milk. Human milk has always been and always will be the best food for human babies.

Babies and airports

Today, it is a common travesty of human justice and decency that parents are frequently forced to throw away an infant's bottle of milk at an airport security checkpoint. I have seen security attendants force parents to put a full bottle of milk through the x-ray machines. They are told it is low-dose x-ray, so it is not harmful. These poor misguided souls are suffering exposure themselves as they stand for hours next to the machines where a sign is visibly posted stating "Danger X-rays—Keep Back." The x-rayed food products are contaminated with radioactive ions. Also, low level radiation has been proven to cause cancer when embryos and infants are exposed to x-irradiation. Dr. Brian MacMahon of the School of Public Health at Harvard University, Dr. Alice Stewart, head of the Department of Preventive Medicine at Oxford University in England, and

Dr. E. B. Lewis of the California Institute of Technology all agree and conclude that low-dose radiation (such as radiation fallout and airport x-ray machines) is as damaging as high dose medical x-ray exposure. Furthermore, the cancer causing effects of radiation are cumulative. That means repeated exposure increases the degree of damage to human tissues.

It was further stated that the fetus in the uterus is hundreds or thousands of times more sensitive to radiation than anyone would have ever suspected. My question is are you willing to take a chance that your baby could be harmed or genetically damaged or even die a horrible death due to cancer? The government told us to just say no—to drugs. So let's just say no to radiation exposure. Refuse to let your baby's bottle of milk or your baby be x-rayed. It is purely a form of tyranny and subjugation of human rights to expose your child to potential cancer-causing ions.

If you think this is just nonsense, then recall that CAT scans so commonly used in hospitals for so long were found to be equal to one hundred chest x-rays. Since they are so dangerous, they are now being used on our luggage and personal belongings—a convenient new market for these machines. All materials retain radioactive ions, and the negative effects increase as the x-rays are done repeatedly. Also, keep in mind that ultrasound so commonly used to view unborn infants has been proven to be dangerous. Therefore, if you are so trusting to think that everything that is being done to you is for your health and safety—think again—and just say no.

Be aware that any food, water, or anything else for sale in an airport has been x-rayed. I saw big tubs of ice cream being run through the x-ray machines with the luggage. The big brouhaha over no bottles of milk, water, or personal items is a contrived method to increase sales in airport stores. Remember, there you are a trapped audience until that plane gets off the ground. Again, let your money speak and boycott anything (or anyone) that is damaging to you or your babies.

All of this is an unnecessary inconvenience and even a danger to the health of the public. Remember, radiation is cumulative. In other words, it builds up and stays in the tissues and affects the cells adversely. The young are always so much more susceptible to any toxin or damaging exposure.

If these airport tactics were so important, then why do they miss so much? It was just reported that a six-month-old kitten crawled into a bag and was shipped 1300 miles. To make matters worse, the bag was mistakenly picked up by another traveler. When he arrived home and opened the bag, the kitten jumped out and hid under the bed. He admitted to screaming at the top of his lungs. Fortunately, the kitten had on a collar with a telephone number, and she made her way back home. Who knows what effect irradiation and lack of oxygen has had on that kitten. Yet, if these inspections are so almighty important, why didn't they find her in the bag? If anyone was intent on destruction, it would be accomplished somehow. All of this is an infringement on our physical health and personal rights. It is obvious that infants and the elderly in wheelchairs are not dangerous terrorists. Yet, they are searched, wanded, and felt-up like they are the most dangerous criminals. Actually, they are the most vulnerable and unable to voice a complaint against such treatment. These invasive requirements are merely fear tactics to keep the masses compliant and subservient to undue power and authority.

Summary: what should babies eat?

Infants should be fed milk. They should be fed human milk. No formula can replace mother's milk no matter what manufacturers and others say. For nine months this fragile creature has been on a life support system within the mother. The infant's tissues recognize the nourishment from the mother and use it readily and successfully for growth and development. Plus, a baby does not have an established immune system, and mother's milk provides protection until the child's own system is established enough to handle any invaders.

During the first feeding breast milk prepares the new digestive system to function properly, and it assists the bowels to begin working and moving out any waste matter. Ideally, nursing should begin within the first hour of birth. Human milk changes consistency to support the needs of the child. It becomes quite rich after the first watery stage, and this provides intense nourishment that is specific and appropriate for the infant's physical welfare.

All of the components of human milk have never been totally identified, so no formula could be exactly the same. Also, it is in the form of predigested nutrients, and no formula is so easily digested and assimilated. Human milk is structurally different than animal milk. For instance, it is rich in fat for the following reasons: fat is necessary for the development of the brain, retina, nervous system, and skin; it is a major source of calories, providing more than twice the energy potential of protein and carbohydrates; it is a carrier for the fat soluble vitamins; and it is needed in the form of cholesterol to make vitamin D. Protein is next. Quality and digestibility are main concerns. There are about 10 to 12 grams per liter of protein in breast milk. Protein is most important for cellular and tissue development. Breast milk supplies two forms of protein: between 60% to 70% is in the form of whey protein, and the remainder is casein. Whey protein is most digestible, and animal milk is much higher in casein which causes digestive upset in infants. Substances, such as lactoferrin, alpha-lactalbumin, albumin, hormones, enzymes, immunoglobulins, and growth factors, are in the proper balance in human whey material. They are not available in animal milk or formula. Finally, carbohydrate is needed for energy and is supplied in the form of lactose, also known as milk sugar. It accounts for about 40% of the energy requirement. Other vital elements are also needed. Minerals must be plentiful such as calcium and magnesium for bones and teeth formation, iron for the blood, and zinc for protein assimilation. Vitamins must be available for their specific purposes that are essential for development of the child. Breast milk from vegetarian/vegan mothers may be low or totally deficient in B_{12} and vitamin A. Both are mandatory for mother and child and must be added to the diet or supplemented in some way.

Growth is greatest during this early phase of life and the changes are dramatic. Only human milk can provide exactly what a human infant needs. Yet, the mother must be careful to get the appropriate nourishment to sustain her health and her baby's well-being.

Babies should be breast-fed a minimum of six months. Studies have determined that babies nourished with breast milk for more than seven months had higher IQs. In general they are happier and healthier, and the immune system is better developed. The sucking action strengthens the jaw, and future teeth will more likely be straight and stronger. They swallow less air, and colic is not as common. Of course, the bonding that occurs between the infant and mother is of utmost importance as well.

More women are breast-feeding their babies now than in the past 50 years. Around 70% are doing so. Yet, I saw a young woman on television recently preaching that formula supplied more nutrients than breast milk, and it gave her so much more freedom. Unfortunately, her child will suffer the consequences. Bottle-feeding was a fad in the 1960s, and it doesn't need to be revived.

Human milk is so important for babies that breast milk banks are now available in California, British Columbia, Texas, Iowa, Michigan, Indiana, Ohio, North Carolina, Massachusetts, and Colorado. This began because sick or premature infants are 10 times more likely to have severe digestive disasters when they are fed formula rather than breast milk. In California alone over 30 neonatal intensive care units use human breast milk. Of course, the milk is tested to be sure it is free of disease-producing viruses or bacteria.

Even wet nurses are beginning to become popular again, mainly for working mothers and women who are unable to produce milk. However, it is very expensive, but services providing wet nurses are available in some areas.

People are always excited to start feeding the baby some kind of food. Especially if the baby cries during the night, many people will start feeding the infant cereal to help it sleep longer. It was also once customary for the doctors to give the baby paregoric, a strong narcotic, to make baby sleep. Neither of these is desirable. If the baby is crying, it may need a longer feeding or it may need more milk than is available. As mentioned before mother's tea, black seed, and fenugreek may be beneficial to increase milk production.

Mother's diet should be organic, well-balanced with vegetables, fruit, grains, and healthy protein sources. Food supplements from organic, wild, and raw whole food sources are usually required depending on the quality and quantity of food ingested. Many young mothers want to lose weight quickly and skimp on desirable foods, which provide high sources of nutrients. Their bodies suffer and so do the babies, since lactation can be physically depleting. Human milk provides only what is available. Moreover, it cannot be overemphasized that while nursing the diet should be free of alcohol, chocolate, coffee and tea, sugar, refined foods, refined/hydrogenated oils and fats, fried foods, chemicals, pesticides, herbicides, and food additives. That is why organic food which is always richer in nutrients and mostly free of chemicals, pesticides, and herbicides will be more beneficial. The more the nursing mother sticks to this way of eating, the healthier, stronger, and happier she and the baby will be.

Most infants are ready for baby food when they are around six months old. Some may be ready at four months, yet breast milk only is perfectly complete for the first year. It basically is up to the mother and child to determine what is desired and needed. It is easier and more economical to feed only the breast milk, as long as the infant is growing and thriving. It also means that the baby's immune system may be stronger, since it is unchallenged by new foods.

There are some do's and don'ts when determining what is healthy and beneficial and what is not. The following should never be given to babies and toddlers:

• beer or other sources of alcohol
• soda pop/soft drinks

- sugar
- white flour/ white bread
- candy/chocolate
- refined food
- tea and coffee
- chemical additives/food dyes
- artificial sweeteners
- pesticide/herbicide contaminated food
- sugared cereals
- nitrated meats-hot dogs/lunch meat
- white rice
- junk food and/or deep-fried food
- genetically modified food

I have seen people give terrible things to infants just to have a laugh at the faces that they make. Not only is this a challenge to their fragile systems, but it can develop early on addictions to substances that will only do harm. If it seems fanatical to say never use sugar and other sweets, then consider this. Obesity and diabetes are rampant among children today. If they don't develop a taste for junk that has no nourishment for their bodies, they will not be addicted to it. Their systems are so much smaller that it doesn't take much to have a toxic load of alcohol, chemicals, or even sugar.

In the beginning the preponderance of a child's diet is mainly fruit and vegetables. Due to small body size and faster metabolisms pesticide/herbicide residues on these foods are highly toxic to children, especially babies and toddlers. The organophosphates (pesticide) so commonly used cause a vast amount of damage, especially to developing nervous systems. Damaged children are then treated with drugs to calm them down or speed them up.

This truly is a time of toxic chemical overload for most everyone. The U.S. National Academy of Science found that by age 5 children acquire around 35% of their lifetime exposure to carcinogenic pesticides. Furthermore, in 2004 the Environmental Working Group found cord blood contained 287 toxic substances. Of these toxic substances 180 are proven to cause cancer in humans and animals, 217 cause damage to brain tissue and the nervous system, and 208 activate birth defects and abnormal development in animals. It is time to stop following the commonly accepted model. Being aware of better choices and making an individual effort to stop these practices by refusing to support them monetarily are required actions for everyone.

Unfortunately, most items in grocery stores do not qualify to be fed to babies and toddlers or anyone else. Certainly, organic fresh fruit and vegetables are the foods of choice. Steam the vegetables and puree them in a blender. Blend the fresh fruit in a blender, or mash it with a fork. Feed the little one immediately so that the vitamins are intact. Avoid grains, since they are mostly refined and usually stale. If you use grains or rice, buy them whole and as fresh as possible. Soak them over night in clean water at room temperature. Then simmer covered for about 30 minutes or until soft enough to eat. When the toddler is ready for meat, start with a bit of blended organic chicken or turkey. It is cheaper to feed the little one good healthy food that is easy to make than to buy the pre-made type. It is fresher, more nutritious, and doesn't compromise the taste buds of the child. Jarred food should be used only when traveling or when other options are not available. Some jarred foods have been found to contain dangerous levels of fluoride. Still others contain monosodium glutamate, a neurotoxin.

Some people think they cannot cook. Yet, it is so easy the baby could do it, if it could stand up and control a blender. There are some rules to follow. First, wash the hands. Hands should *always* be cleaned after changing a diaper and before preparing food. Many people forget to do this, because they have never developed this important hygiene habit. Baby poop can be just as dangerous as that from any other human or creature. For example, a woman was preparing dinner, when her infant developed diarrhea. She failed to wash her hands after changing diapers. Let's just say her guests suffered great anguish as a result of food poisoning. Secondly, wash the food. Even if it is supposedly pre-washed, don't believe it. Vegetables especially can carry germs such as e-coli, salmonella, and parasites. Such exposure is a painful experience for the baby and the caretaker as well. Third, lightly scrape or peel the food if necessary, and remove any seeds or membranes. Fourth, don't overcook the food. Steaming keeps the vitamins and minerals in the food. Thus, they are not lost in the cooking water. Fifth, have fun and get creative. Use as much raw, soft food as possible such as avocados and bananas. The internet may be helpful especially for anyone who has had little cooking experience. On YouTube there are videos with mothers demonstrating how to prepare food for babies, toddlers, and various ages of children. This is one benefit of the information age.

Baby/Toddler recipes

¼ boiled potato
2 tablespoons organic whole milk (preferably non-pasteurized goat or sheep milk) or potato water

Mash the potato with a fork and mix in milk or cooking water from the boiled potato until smooth. If necessary, add more liquid to make it creamy and easy to eat. A teaspoon of butter NOT margarine may be added as well. Butter is a good source of vitamin A. Remember, for freshness add 1 or 2 drops of wild oregano oil in extra virgin olive oil per quart of unpasteurized milk. Whip it into the milk. This amount does not alter the flavor.

1 carrot or sweet potato
2 or 3 tablespoons vegetable broth

Scrape the carrot or peel the sweet potato and wash it. Cut it into sticks. Steam or simmer the sticks in a small amount of water until semi soft. The carrot or sweet potato can be mashed with the liquid added to make a thin purée, and this is best for babies. Use the sticks as finger food for the toddler. Note: all vegetables such as squash, broccoli, peas, green beans, etc. can be steamed, baked, or simmered until tender and then mashed or blended. For essential fatty acids ½ teaspoon of raw sacha inchi oil, pumpkinseed oil, sesame seed oil, or Alaskan sock-eye salmon oil may be added to the mashed vegetables. This will supply the much-needed essential fatty acids.

6 to 8 organic blueberries and strawberries

Rinse with cold water and serve whole for the older toddler. They are perfect finger foods.

½ apple
3 tablespoons fresh orange juice

Wash and peel the apple. Grate the apple, and mix with 3 tablespoons of fresh orange juice. Feed the raw apple sauce to the toddler immediately. Baked apple puréed or apple sauce may be given to the six-month-old baby.

¼ small raw avocado
1 to 2 inches of ripe banana (optional)

Wash, peel, and mash the avocado with a fork. This is a highly nourishing fruit for the baby as early as four months old and for the toddler too. It is rich in many vitamins and minerals and supports growth and development, especially for the central nervous system and brain. It is far superior as a first food than refined cereals. It can be combined with a small piece of mashed banana as well. Mashed banana is a good first food along with the avocado.

¼ lb. chicken or turkey breast

Cut cleaned turkey or chicken breast into cubes, and place meat in a covered baking dish. Sprinkle with 3 or 4 tablespoons of water. Bake in 350°F oven until tender. Blend until totally smooth, adding any juice left from the baking. Other meat, such as organic lamb and beef, can be prepared the same way. Do not use pork, bacon, or ham as baby food. Puréed meat can be introduced to the 7- to 10-month old baby. Organic meat prepared for the family can be puréed for the toddlers. Add meat juice or water to the meat and blend.

1 organic egg yolk

Soft boil or poach an egg. Peel a soft-boiled egg, and remove the yolk. Remove the white from a poached egg. Mash the egg yolk only. It can be eaten plain or with vegetables. It is rich in vitamin A and B-vitamins. Start baby on organic egg yolk at around 8 months. Watch for any allergic reaction, if the baby is allergy prone.

Eating should be a delightful experience. It is a social time, and a time to nourish the body with healthy nourishing food. The food must be fresh and the best that is available. It is acceptable to freeze extra portions, but it should be used within three months. However, fresh is always best to maintain the highest level of nutrient quality and fuel value.

Never use a microwave oven for food preparation. It destroys the vitamins, damages the proteins, and oxidizes the fat. It ionizes the food as well.

It is always better to eat small quantities of excellent food than huge quantities of bad food. Many Americans eat far too much. Yet, the food may be so deficient in nutrients, that they never feel full. They also never feel good.

Food has a huge emotional impact. What is learned in childhood as being good, tasty, or appropriate will usually be remembered and practiced throughout a lifetime. That is why the fast food restaurants make a great effort to attract young children. Then, they have customers for life. Once the taste buds are corrupted by sugar and deep-fried foods, as well as refined and packaged treats, the desire for wholesome, healthy food is decreased. Never doubt that this has cost the American nation dearly in relation to health, work capacity, and financial stability as well.

This book is designed to build understanding and knowledge. The messages may not always be popular, but the future of this nation and, actually, the entire world is dependent upon making better choices.

Chapter Three

Building a Super Child

Isn't it desirable to want a strong and healthy child who is calm, yet attentive, intelligent, and alert? Isn't it important that a child has a resistant immune system, so that he/she does not readily pick up colds, flu, other infections and various diseases? What are parents willing to do to make this happen?

Children do have likes and dislikes even as babies. They may have food sensitivities or just don't like the taste, texture, or smell of certain substances. It is not uncommon to be able to tolerate food or even supplements one day and not another. Regarding a food supplement Dr. Lendon Smith suggested smelling it before consuming the daily dose. If it smells good or there is no apparent smell, which is generally the rule, take it. If it smells bad, do not take it. That is a simple little rule to help sort out what the body chemistry can handle that day. Yes, even with the same supplements the smell may vary from day to day. When this is done with children, it is not a good idea to tell them that they don't have to take it if it smells bad. Guess what their answers most likely will be unless it is a sugar-laden synthetic vitamin/mineral concoction that tastes like candy. They need to be carefully trained from birth to abhor the most destructive substances they can eat, and that means refined sugars and artificial sweeteners. Refined sugars and artificial sweeteners are addictive substances. Raw, unprocessed honey and raw yacon syrup are good choices, when a sweetener is desired. Otherwise, refined sweeteners should be avoided like the plague. There is not a single benefit from eating sugar. There isn't even a benefit of bringing happiness, since the taste is soon gone and strong cravings remain. Besides, most B complex vitamins, which I call the happiness vitamins, are destroyed. Who needs that? If parents are hooked on sugar, that doesn't mean they need to expose their progeny to the addiction. The physical, mental, and emotional damage that these substances cause are not worth it. Ask any reformed sugarholic, if you can find one. It is not an act of kindness and love to reward with sugar, because obesity, dental caries, bone loss, diabetes, depression, dermatitis, and acne are just a few of the actual "rewards" of eating such addictive substances.

Vitamins and health

Vitamins are minute substances found in unrefined food that cause a person to thrive with good health. When they are deficient, mysterious diseases seem to appear. Scurvy, rickets, beri-beri, and pellagra were once thought to be caused by microbes. It wasn't until 1911 that Casimir Funk coined the word vita-amine when an extract from rice polishings amazingly cured beri-beri. This finally opened some minds, and soon scientists discovered other natural substances which cured previously mysterious diseases.

Most research and discoveries in the field of nutrition were accomplished after the turn of the twentieth century. At that time (unlike today) there was government grant money dedicated to studying the unknown natural chemicals in food. Over twenty vitamins were isolated and their purposes identified. Today, the nutritional quality of food is being altered for the worse. To complete the insult, toxic artificial chemicals are also being added. In addition, unscrupulous researchers are relentlessly destroying the real food of nature, which was designed by our creator to nourish and build our bodies. This, of course, is the genetic alteration of plants to make them patentable. Thus, all seeds and all food produced on this earth can be controlled by a few major sources. This is dangerous for many reasons.

Today, there are still many powerful natural agents in food that are unnamed and unknown. No one even knows what they can actually do for the body. Now unless there is a potential for patenting and major financial gain, there is little independent research and not a lot of interest in new discoveries for health improvement. Without government funding and with minimal independent research actively being conducted, growth and development of preventive health and healing continue to be inhibited. It is important to support those who have integrity. This is especially true when their efforts are focused upon improving preventive healthcare and providing this valuable information for the welfare of all of mankind.

Dr. Ron Paul is a man of such integrity. He is a licensed medical doctor and a United States Congressman. For over 23 years he has voted for the rights of the people of the United States according to the Constitution. This should include the right to be educated. Education enables people to be better equipped to make intelligent choices for the food that they eat and the supplements that they take to maintain health and well-being. Currently, the American public is denied these freedoms and rights. However, Paul has introduced bills HR2117, HR2717, HR3394, and HR3395 to try to obtain health freedom, personal choice, and a balance of power. To have the right to know about nutritive values, healing properties of food, and valuable information on nutritional supplements, everyone must contact their representatives and senators in Washington, D.C. *Do this constantly.* For the benefit of humanity everyone who values freedom of choice must demand that these bills are passed. We must keep demanding until they are. The Citizens for Health had a response of over 4000 people who contacted their representatives in three days concerning these bills, but that was certainly not enough. All people who are concerned about human welfare must make their voices heard. Civil liberties of all citizens should be a main concern of those in power.

Fortunately, even if the focus is on only what information is currently available, it is possible to enjoy long and healthy lives. Food that is rich in the known nutrients will also be rich in those unknown cofactors, which contribute to good health. Healthy eating is essential for all people and future generations. Children must grow up strong, stable, and intelligent so they can find their appropriate paths in this world. It is a moral obligation to do the research and protect them from those who have no interest but financial gain and unlimited power. Every dollar spent is a vote. A vote may be cast for good, or it can be cast for bad depending on what is purchased. It is always wise to remember that people still have the buying power. Organic food, which is NON-genetically engineered, is the best choice for everyone.

These genetically corrupted foods, known as GMOs, have been forced into the marketplace. Those same foods should at least have required labeling so that people can make intelligent decisions to buy or not to buy. However, with all the strict government policing and regulations that are constantly increasing and restricting our personal freedoms, it can only be that corporate coercion reigns over these government agencies. This is evident, since there is no requirement to list GMOs on the labels of food products, even though the public has repeatedly requested that this information be made available. GMOs even contaminate many of the food supplements.

Actually, the first sales of canola oil were transacted by the health food industry. Virtually all canola that is not organic is genetically modified. Look at the food labels in all stores, including the health food stores, to determine if canola oil is a listed ingredient. If so, is it organic? This means that everyone needs to be aware and must conduct the necessary homework to stay informed. Individual and family protection is the main purpose of this effort. Since it is not required to list GMOs on labels, the only option is to buy organic, fresh from the farm, or food labeled non-GMO. However, there is another scary fact, and that is a food may be grown organically from genetically modified seed. Once again this proves that labeling should be required and enforced, if protection of the public is really of any concern. There is no evidence that genetically modified foods are safe and fit for human consumption. No appropriate testing has been done, nor could research determine all the possible long-range damage. The damage to human tissue takes time, although youngsters and the elderly are the most easily and seriously challenged from the beginning. Other countries demand that all GMOs are listed on their food labels. All informed people refuse to buy them. Many countries refuse to buy products from the United States due to GMO status.

Furthermore, in countries where people are starving, their leaders wisely refuse such contamination for their hungry masses, even if it is donated.

If you do not think this is important, do your research. This is a worldwide crisis, as biotech companies are taking away seeds from people who have grown their own plants and seeds for hundreds of years. Then, they are forced to use seeds that have been horribly corrupted. Most importantly, this corruption changes the structure of plants, and it is forever so. It is merely for control and power, because these genetically engineered plants are proven to be less prolific than original seeds and hybrids. That means the altered seeds yield less than the original heirloom seeds and their resulting plants that have been grown for hundreds of years. If this continues, world hunger, which is massively on the increase, will reach a crisis point. Those who control the food (seeds) and water ultimately control the world.

Food is the major source of nourishment. Therefore, it should provide energy, growth factors, vitamins, minerals, antioxidants, enzymes, fiber, and more. Even when food is unprocessed, it is rarely available at the peak of its perfection. Nor is food ever served immediately, which is obviously ideal. Totally fresh, healthy food is like no other. I have eaten fish caught in a pristine wilderness lake, and within minutes it was cleaned and then cooked over a campfire. Wild berries picked fresh off the vine taste excitingly different from the cultivated kinds. Anything picked green, shipped for thousands of miles, and artificially ripened cannot compare taste-wise or nutrition-wise. There is nothing comparable to the taste and nutritional density of freshly picked and prepared food.

While living in Germany, I would occasionally go out to eat at the little family-owned gasthaus inns. Sometimes you could watch the proprietor walk out to the organic garden in back, carefully pick the best of the salad makings, and prepare them fresh. The mouthwatering taste of a large variety of organic herbs and vegetables grown from heirloom seeds (the original and unaltered seeds, which provide the most luscious taste and greatest food value) can only be imagined. When food is prepared this fresh, the textures, colors, and flavors are to be savored. Furthermore, the healthy nutrients directly influenced by the sun, the rain, and the air are at their peak. That is how food is meant to be eaten. Long shipping times, poor storage facilities, exposure to artificial light, excessively high or low temperatures, spraying with chemicals, waxing or gassing, x-ray exposure and any other improper handling all affect the degree of nourishment available in the food and the resulting energy that the cells of the body can ultimately receive. Also, prolonged cooking readily destroys nutrients such as the delicate vitamins. Then, most of the few remaining vitamins and minerals are thrown out with the cooking water. Eating the largest proportion of food as fresh as possible in the raw state is always best for the entire family.

It must not be forgotten that there are additional toxins due to constant bombing overseas. This planet has an enclosed atmosphere which encircles the globe. The radioactive depleted uranium from the bombs is misted into the air. The contamination reaches every part of this planet. Even the most remote areas, the ice caps, and the jungles are contaminated by man-made poisons and irradiation. The effects of radioactivity are devastating, especially for the young, and it is a contamination that lasts for thousands of years. The only solution is that it must stop immediately for the sake of all life on the planet.

The best that can be done is filter all household water and eat organic food. Does it seem as if there is no time to prepare healthy meals? Small powerful blenders, such as the Bullet Blender or the mighty Vita Mix, are two machines which make great raw baby food, soups, sauces, nut milks, smoothies, and much more. These machines make preparing healthy meals fast and easy, and this delicious food will nourish and strengthen bodies and brains.

Kids need nourishment

Without the proper nourishment there will be failure to thrive. That is why I look on in astonishment at the television programs depicting the poor starving children in Africa who are fed white slimy gruel in the name of ending starvation. While the intensions are surely honorable, the results are largely disruptive. When children are eating a diet of whatever is fast and easy, including goodies they see on television commercials, or they are junk food addicts, they are no better off than starving children in Africa. Because of inadequate diets and genetically altered, nutritionally depleted, sprayed and poisoned food, an increasing number of young people are dying from "unknown causes." This includes babies in cribs and youngsters on the basketball court. Recently, in the Chicago area the school board attempted to mandate heart screenings (EKGs) for children before they are allowed to participate in school activities. This action resulted because of over 300 athletic-related sudden deaths among school age children. This is definitely due to the malnutrition of these children. Even though they may not be suddenly dropping dead, most children are poorly nourished. This is because they are junk food junkies.

As long as they eat such depleted, even poisoned food, they cannot possibly reach their full mental, physical, and, thus, spiritual potential.

While overpopulation seems to be a major concern in the world, if industry continues such dastardly practices, the human race will be at extreme risk for continued degeneration. It is time that everything possible is done to protect the sanctity of the planet, human life, and the strength and integrity of future generations. That is why knowledge is so valuable. However, this takes a certain amount of effort and research. The greatest achievement on this planet requires that the majority of people adopt the willingness to cooperate for the highest good. As people learn and understand more it is easier to change existing habits for better food choices and healthier life practices. This chapter is dedicated to providing that knowledge and understanding.

WATER SOLUBLE VITAMINS

Water soluble vitamins readily mix with body fluids and are able to cross the blood-brain barrier, which is designed to block toxic substances. Thus, these vitamins in the natural form are easily recognized and are a benefit to brain and body functions. Then, they are quickly carried to the receptor sites, where they are needed. Natural sources of these vitamins from unprocessed organic food are best, because they stay in the body longer and are better absorbed and utilized. This has been proven by many research studies. Most multiple vitamins are a combination of water and fat soluble vitamins, but they are most likely from synthetic sources. Even if it says on the bottle "all natural" or even "food source" it is always best to determine the actual content and where it was derived. If it is above a few milligrams, it is most likely synthetic or partially synthetic. When people see 500 mg per serving on labels, they think they are getting more for their money, because a natural product may show only a low milligram dose. However, they are not getting a value. Those who are informed demand a food-based supplement. The best source of nourishment is always from pesticide-free, nutrient-dense food supplements. There is a nutrient-dense food supplement containing rice polish/bran and crushed flax as the main ingredients, which may be added to smoothies, cereal, or your favorite recipes. This is an example of a real and natural source of vitamins and minerals. Most tablets, capsules, and chewy things are likely not the ideal.

The B complex vitamins and vitamin C are the known water soluble vitamins. That means that vitamins B and C, which are not readily used by the body, are rapidly lost. Therefore, keep in mind that every time little "Alex" or "Alexis" uses the potty or comes in hot and sweaty or cries those big crocodile tears, he/she is losing vitamins. For superior health in both children and adults, all water soluble nutrients need to be replenished daily. In most countries, including the United States, this is not happening.

B complex includes thiamine (B_1), riboflavin (B_2), niacin (B_3), pantothenic acid (B_5), pyridoxine (B_6), vitamin B_{12}, folic acid, biotin, choline, inositol, and PABA. All B vitamins have specific functions and purposes. However, many of them are found in the same food sources and seem to have similar benefits. That led scientists to believe that the various B vitamins must work synergistically. For best results all the water soluble vitamins should be consumed in some kind of fresh food every day. Thus, even the unknown, unnamed factors which are needed for physical and mental health will be ingested and will be beneficial for maintaining health.

There are many cases of childhood malnutrition today. Many young mothers do not know how to cook and have no interest in learning. For example, a teenage mother, who is pregnant with her second child, consumes mainly pizza or some other fast food every day. She feeds the first baby pizza or fast food as well. The child now has frequent seizures, and his lips and skin turn blue. When the seizures occur, she calls an ambulance and rushes the child to the hospital. The doctors do tests and say he probably will grow out of it by the time he is around six years old. No other solutions are offered, and never do they inquire about the child's diet.

Fortunately, a nutrition expert told this young mother to eat better and to take whole food nutritional supplements for the developing baby. Then, she was informed that her son must eat healthy food, or his degeneration would continue. Now, he is at least eating organic eggs, orange juice, bananas, yogurt, and some other fresh foods. Also, he is taking a tablespoon of fresh Polar-source wild Alaskan salmon oil, plus a royal jelly combination formula full of protein, B vitamins, and other important nutrients. Then, at bedtime he takes a probiotic especially made for children. At first the young woman tried to hide the supplements in food and in orange juice. However, he was quite happy to take all of the supplements without any cover-up or fuss. After changing his diet for the better and adding the nutritional supplements, no more seizures occurred. Also, the flabby fat has disappeared, and he is growing taller and stronger. No doubt, the toddler will continue to respond to the better diet and nutritional supplements as long as these necessary nutrients remain available. It cannot be emphasized enough that for fine physical health and appearance children, as well as the entire family, should enjoy the best possible diet and supplements.

If fast food is an occasional treat, then, hopefully, it won't be too harmful. Yet, a couple lost their ten-year-old son after eating fast food. The young boy took a bath about an hour after eating a food dye-laden concoction. For the first time ever he had a seizure while in the bath tub. Sadly, this precious child drowned before anyone could help him. It is not possible to predict such a reaction. Therefore, it is always better to eat whole organic food and beverages, while avoiding all foods that contain chemical additives.

Thiamine (B₁)

Thiamine is commonly known as the morale vitamin, meaning that with an adequate daily intake the well-nourished individual is enthusiastic and full of good spirits. A high morale is always desirable at home, at school, or at play. It's every coach's dream to create and maintain a high morale. This is important, because with good morale, mental fiber, and physical strength, his/her team will always be a winner.

If the consequence of thiamine deficiency is low morale, think of all the implications this could mean. Could there be a connection between all the children who have behavioral problems at home and in school? Are children and adults alike really deficient in drugs as the commercials on television would like for us to believe? Could it possibly be that they are thiamine deficient? Would the millions of depressed people consuming millions of dollars of mind-altering drugs feel better if they just changed their diets for the better and, perhaps, took natural vitamin supplements?

Nearly all school age children are consuming mind-altering substances. This includes sugar as one of the worst offenders. Few if any have adequate thiamine in their diets. Actually, what they eat may destroy whatever thiamine they have. The signs and symptoms are always present, but they are usually not even recognized. The following are some of the symptoms children (and adults as well) may experience when there is a thiamine deficiency.

- neuritis/nerve trouble
- constipation
- subnormal growth
- poor appetite
- chronic fatigue
- racing heart
- degeneration of the heart
- tires easily
- poor memory
- depression
- nausea
- noise sensitivity
- low birth weight
- loss of weight
- overweight
- digestive disturbances
- headaches
- irritability
- chest pain
- crave sugar/starch
- lack of initiative
- confused thinking
- fear
- inability to concentrate
- mental disease
- high pyruvic acid levels
- insect magnet, especially mosquitoes

How thiamine functions in the body

Thiamine has two main functions. The first is energy production. Then, thiamine is necessary for the conversion of acids which develop during energy production. It acts like a coenzyme, since it is helps to convert blood sugar into energy. As energy is produced from blood sugar, there are two acids which are formed. These are pyruvic and lactic acids. Enzymes in combination with thiamine oxidize pyruvic acid. Thus, it is destroyed. Through a different process thiamine is necessary for lactic acid to be converted into glycogen. Glycogen is a type of sugar, which is stored in the liver. Ultimately, it is converted into blood sugar. This is why thiamine deficiency is directly related to blood sugar irregularities.

When the diet is deficient in thiamine, pyruvic and lactic acids accumulate throughout body tissues. These acids are especially prevalent in the brain, nerves, heart, and blood. These irritating substances damage those tissues and reduce the body's energy production. This would account for such symptoms as aches and pains, moodiness and anger, and blood sugar swings. It is common that after strenuous exercise there is a lactic acid buildup in the body. Yet, it is more likely a symptom of thiamine deficiency.

Much of the energy produced from blood sugar is used by the brain as well as the nerves. Needless to say, there is damage to these cells, when the proper nourishment is lacking. Common symptoms are headaches, nervousness, irritability, neuritis, shakiness, nausea, dizziness, and fainting. These symptoms are the body's cry for help.

Further damage occurs as the energy for the digestive processes is impeded. As a result, the stomach contractions are weakened and the digestive juices are not thoroughly mixed with the food. Hydrochloric acid is needed for protein breakdown, but unfortunately, in some people the HCL levels are too low or non-existent. A wave-like action, which causes the movement of ingested food in the intestines, is also more sluggish. The partially digested rotting food stays in the intestines too long, and the waste matter becomes dry and hardens. Constipation and toxicity are the result. This may be the main reason so many children suffer from chronic constipation, especially if it is combined with depression, agitation, and moodiness.

When disruptions occur with digestion, then there is a domino effect. All the other digestive substances, such as bile, pancreatic enzymes, the digestive enzymes which act as ferments, and intestinal fluids, are diminished. All these substances are vital for good digestion. It has been said that we are what we eat, but that is not altogether true. Actually, we are what we digest. When digestion is impaired, so is the overall health.

How is it possible to determine if a child is suffering from poor digestion? The following are some symptoms, and the more that occur the greater the digestion is impaired.

- burping/belching
- flatulence
- gas pains/ bloating
- stomach problems
- bad breath
- poor appetite
- undigested food in the stool
- smelly stools
- weight loss
- nausea
- constipation
- diarrhea
- vomiting
- poor growth
- weight gain

Thiamine deficiency—cause for obesity

As explained earlier thiamine is necessary for the production of energy. When thiamine is deficient, sweet and starchy foods are only partially converted to energy. This is because there is a lack of important enzymes. Thus, these partially digested substances are stored as fat.

The obese child and adult usually tire quickly and quite literally are lacking in energy due to decreased availability of blood sugar. If they try to exercise, they quickly become breathless and may experience heart palpitations. There is usually a constant craving for sweets, which do provide short bursts of energy. Then, energy levels fall, and the cravings begin again. Sugar is rapidly absorbed without being broken down by enzymes. Ultimately, hypoglycemia (low blood sugar) develops due to flooding the system with sugar. Too much insulin is the result. With overproduction of insulin the cravings are continuous, the weight increases, fatigue and weakness prevent much needed exercise, and the mental state is depressed. This must be corrected, or it is a matter of time before the individual develops diabetes and other serious health problems. Also, all sweets feed fungus. The fungus needs sugar to survive, so the craving becomes almost obsessive. The fungus attacks the thyroid to feed on important nutrients, and this further impairs metabolic function. At this point it is difficult, if not impossible, to lose weight without a carefully planned diet and supplement program.

Mediterranean oil of oregano (wild, handpicked) is invaluable for purging fungus. This purge helps with normalizing thyroid function. Now it is possible to lose weight. As strength and stamina improve with weight loss, an exercise and deep breathing program is mandatory. When the thyroid is sluggish, oxygen intake in the cells is poor. Low oxygen levels also impede weight loss. The cells need the oxygen to burn fuel. While many factors contribute to the increasing incidence of childhood and, ultimately, adult obesity, a number of diseases arise from poor nutrition and obesity. Yet, omitting sugar and junk food are the first steps for preventing this. Sugar and junk food must be replaced by whole wild or organic food. Vital nutrients from healthy food and whole food supplements help to eliminate most of the serious symptoms and even curtail disease.

Heart damage and beri-beri

Thiamine deficiency doesn't just mean that an individual will be in a bad mood and, perhaps, have problems getting along with others. The consequences are far more dire. Researchers have determined that the heart is the first organ which is damaged from thiamine deficiency. At first a thiamine deficiency slows the heartbeat. Then, as the deficiency is prolonged and the severity increases, the heart muscle becomes irritated. This is because of the build-up of pyruvic and lactic acids. This results in a racing heartbeat. If the deficiency is not addressed and only drugs are administered for the symptoms, heart failure is the result.

Fluid collection around the heart is another common symptom caused by a lack of this nutrient. This is actually a symptom of the wet form of beri-beri. Wet and dry beri-beri are much the same, but the wet form means that there is edema, while with the dry form there is none. Other symptoms for both forms are chronic constipation, loss of feeling, loss of motor function and muscle degeneration, or, finally, paralysis of the lower extremities due to systemic inflammation of the nerves.

Modern arrogance would lead us to believe that (wet and dry) beri-beri is an old-fashioned disease of the past and that no one has such a problem today. This is false. First of all, doctors and clinicians have studied little to no nutrition. Therefore, they fail to recognize what they are seeing, and only the obvious symptoms are treated. Constipation is the earliest symptom of subclinical (early onset) disease. Yet, this is treated with various kinds of laxatives. These further reduce the natural movement of the intestines and increase the flaccidity (loss of tone) of the bowel walls. Throughout the United States people are experiencing all stages of sub-clinical beri-beri. While we have the most food in the world, it is among the worst nutritionally. The most common victims are children and adults who consume large amounts of refined food such as white bread, white rice, and sugar.

Constipation is the number one complaint for children across the nation. So many children start their day with sugar over sugar-coated refined cereal, plus white flour fried donuts, sweet rolls or candy bars, and artificially flavored sugar-sweetened juices or sodas. Lunch is something like white flour pizza or mad meat hot dogs and more sodas or sugary tea drinks. Finally, they end it with more sugar-contaminated, refined TV dinners, cookies, and just maybe a glass of "skim milk." There is virtually no thiamine or anything else of value available in this mess called food. If there is any thiamine, it would be in a synthetic form such as thiamine hydrochloride. It is probably added as a so-called food fortifier to the refined white flour. There may be a small amount in the ground pork guts mixed in with the hot dogs. Thiamine hydrochloride is so difficult to digest that out of 100 milligrams consumed only around 10 milligrams are absorbed by the body. Then, absorption only occurs if the individual's digestion is functioning superbly. Needless to say, this is a rarity. Also, sugar destroys thiamine, so children who are sugar addicts have a severe daily thiamine deficit. No wonder they are hyperactive terrors or hypoactive depressives, who have a bowel movement with great effort—maybe—once a week. Thus, with decaying food and chemicals festering in their bowels, children suffer from headaches, stomachaches, bad breath and gas.

One young boy who was fed happy meals consistently from the time he grew teeth now suffers from mega-colon. This means that the bowel swells and enlarges due to poor nutrition. In his case this led to bowel incontinence and weight gain. Parents, grandparents, and others must be made aware that they are inflicting these conditions on the children they love by denying them healthy food. These parents and grandparents normally have the same health complaints as the children. It isn't difficult to guess why they do. It is because all family members eat the same depleted foods.

The signs and symptoms are not usually hereditary, but the eating and living habits frequently are. Generation after generation, people follow the same familial habits and suffer from the same diseases and health complaints. Instead of recommending an increasing number of drugs a responsible healthcare provider must be informed about the body's function and needs. This is in relation to nutrition, exercise, and the avoidance of all things toxic. The practitioners must, therefore, adequately inform those who come to them for counsel to alter their life-threatening habits.

It is a terrible shame that absolute poisons, such as synthetic sweeteners and over 9000 other deleterious chemicals, are readily offered to the unsuspecting public. Unfortunately, many people truly believe that government agencies protect them from dangerous substances. The lobbyists from big businesses manipulate information in both the House and Senate, and the laws are passed in their favor. This is an example of criminal capitalism. Change can occur only by being informed about what is truly useful for the individual, the family, and the rest of the human race. Then, careful and responsible spending of any discretionary income (the paycheck) for beneficial products can make a huge difference. If useless and possibly harmful products are not purchased, they cannot last in the marketplace. Honesty and decency help keep everything in balance.

There is also another powerful way to achieve a higher consciousness. One of the most effective methods to create positive change is to make a focus board. Use a heavy white paper about three feet by three feet. Place it where it is most easily visible on a wall or door. Kids love this project, and it builds family bonding. Systematically, find every picture that explicitly represents a better way of life. The best pictures represent whatever is beneficial personally as well as for the human race. Glue the pictures onto the focus board. Place full attention on this focus board for a period of time throughout the day and night. Be excited about these changes for the better. Talk about positive happenings, and avoid negative and destructive actions. At least make sure there is enough thiamine in the diet to keep family morale high. Thoughts are power. A lack of thiamine leads to negativity. An abundance of this nutrient in the diet creates positive behavior and a high morale.

Thiamine sources and requirements

Natural thiamine from commercial food is not commonly available. Most all refined foods contain virtually none. When it became evident that the boxes the food came in had more food value (fiber, at least) than the actual refined product, food fortification began. However, out of 25 or so nutrients removed by processing only six or seven are added back to the food. What's more, these are synthetic. Synthetic vitamins are not the same, since they are actually the mirror image of the natural vitamins. Plus, they are made from substances, such as coal tar and oil residues, which are inedible. Thus, the different energy of the synthetic substances confuses the body. Thus, the body interprets them differently than natural vitamins. It seems to use just barely enough of the synthetics as is possible to survive. Natural vitamins—even water soluble ones—stay in the body for a longer time than the synthetic and are more readily absorbed. In the cells they are also more effectively used.

The best source of natural thiamine is nutritional yeast. However, fungal diseases are common, and some yeasts may cause a reaction. Fungus grows when there is an excessive intake of refined carbohydrates and antibiotics. If babies do not have yeast in their bodies when they are born, they surely will have it by the time they are six weeks old. For serious deficiencies nutritional yeast is still worth trying, unless symptoms such as gas, bloating, burping, itching, and bowel disturbances become apparent. It is generally available through health food stores. However, some sources of yeast are better than others, since some may be GMO contaminated. Perhaps the best nutritional yeast currently available is from torula yeast. This form of yeast is also rich in other B vitamins and amino acids.

Other good sources (organic is best) are wheat germ, rice bran and oat bran, almonds, Brazil nuts, sunflower seeds, pecans, carob, and cashews. Other fair sources are eggs, fish, and some vegetables such as avocado, asparagus, turnips, peas, legumes, and some beans.

Today, with the food so depleted and refined and stress levels at an all time high, the majority of people are likely to be deficient. Yet, overall the best common food source is rice bran and polish. These are dense sources of B complex, which most everyone needs.

Food fortifiers from all natural foods that are rich in nutrients are excellent sources of thiamine. One of the best contains rice bran, rice polish, and red sour grape powder. Children and adults love this in shakes. This nutrient-rich product can be added to casseroles, soups, and salads. It makes a delicious breading or coating. As a nutrient booster it is important to add it to homemade pancakes and cookies. It may also be added to juices and smoothies. One recipe that few children can resist is the following:

Berry Berry Good Shake

1 cup organic full fat unsweetened yogurt
1 cup frozen organic berries of choice (do not thaw)
2 tablespoons wild, raw honey or yacon syrup to taste
¼ cup pine nuts (optional—adds protein and makes creamier—or increase to 1/3 cup pine nuts and 1/3 cup of water: use as a replacement for the yogurt
2 tablespoons rice bran/polish with red sour grape powder

Blend in blender or smoothie maker until smooth and creamy. *Some or all of the following optional ingredients may be added to the shake before blending. The more of these options that are used, the more nutritious it is.* These natural food optional ingredients supply more nourishment than multiple vitamins. That also means they are far more beneficial and safer than synthetic, sugar-sweetened pills.

Optional additions to shake:

1   tablespoon Austrian pumpkinseed oil (for essential fatty acids, chlorophyll, phytosterols, and natural vitamin E)

1   dropperful natural-source liquid C (one of the finest sources of liquid natural vitamin C plus co-factors)

1   heaping teaspoonful children's formula royal jelly (pre-digested nutrient-rich natural vitamin, mineral, and amino acid replacement for synthetic multiple vitamins and minerals)

½   ripe frozen banana (freeze with skin, remove skin before blending.) Banana makes a shake creamier and sweeter for the child who has a super sweet tooth.

1   to 3 tablespoons organic sunflower seeds (an excellent source of vitamins, minerals, and proteins—soak seeds overnight in just enough water to cover the seeds before adding to the shake. This will increase digestibility of vitamins and minerals.)

1   tablespoonful raw whole grape powder (terrific source of natural chromium. Research has proven that chromium is necessary for muscle development, the prevention of nearsightedness, and blood sugar control.)

¼   cup melon juice (the taste is quite sweet and almost floral. It is truly delightful, and only a small amount is needed for flavoring. See www.Americanwildfoods.com.)

Place all desired ingredients into a blender and blend on high speed. Stop occasionally and scrape sides to make sure all ingredients are completely processed and mixed. If so desired, add ice chips/cubes to thin and blend until smooth. This is a luscious and nutrient-rich delight. This shake is so filling and so delicious that rarely will children refuse to drink it. This recipe is more than enough to share. Another option is to freeze the remainder for an after school snack in place of ice cream. It is far better to use this shake—especially when the optional items are added—than commercial, sweetened, synthetic vitamin supplements and commercial ice cream full of chemicals. This shake is full of the B vitamins, especially the difficult-to-find natural thiamine. For fussy children who have poor appetites, once they consume this on a regular basis—even a tablespoon a day—their appetites almost always improve. Also, behavior, growth, and overall health are noticeably better.

Why not let the kids help make the shake? Most children like to help and are less picky and finicky when they are involved. They can get creative with the ingredients, as long as it is organic, natural pure food that will help them grow and thrive. It is ideal to premix the ingredients in the blender (except for the frozen berries) the night before and let them sort of "predigest" in the refrigerator. Then, in the morning add the frozen berries and blend. With this method the nutrients are more easily digested and better absorbed. This is nutrition at its finest.

The daily requirement for thiamine varies according to age, size, metabolism, and the amount of carbohydrates consumed. Infants, children, and especially adolescents need thiamine for growth and well-being. For a minimum daily intake infants require 0.6 mg, children need at least 1.0 mg, and adolescents no less than 1.5 mg. Most kids are so depleted from constantly eating a poor, refined food diet that additional thiamine in truly natural wild or organic food supplements is required for good health and behavior. If the child is overweight, the daily requirement increases.

Documented cases have shown some children require therapeutic levels of thiamine. For example, a boy was unable to function physically and mentally until he was given 1500 mg of thiamine daily. While this high amount is an unusual exception due to an inborn error of metabolism, most children require more than the minimum daily requirement, which is the dosage for mere survival.

Sugar and foods, such as white rice as well as other refined carbohydrates, rob the body of nutrients rather than provide them. It is always best to use a thiamine source with some form of natural B complex, since B vitamins work best when used together. The B vitamins are mandatory for growth, performance, and mental balance. Wild and organic foods and food-based supplements are your best choices.

Riboflavin (B₂)

This substance was first detected in milk whey as early as 1897. However, it wasn't called riboflavin until after 1932. It was discovered because of its yellow-green fluorescent pigment. This pigment was found in both plants and animals and rightfully considered a highly important nutrient.

Riboflavin is fairly stable in food, but exposure to light destroys it. Since riboflavin is a water-soluble B vitamin, food containing this nutrient should be cooked in a minimum amount of water. It is fairly heat stable, but it is easily destroyed by irradiation. Today, more and more of our foods are contaminated with radioactive ions from the so-called irradiation preservation process (or contamination at airports where even baby bottles are x-rayed). Also at U.S. ports of entry overseas shipments are irradiated. This destructive energy is harmful, especially for little children. The loss of nutrients alone from this corrupted exposure is deplorable. Not only is riboflavin totally destroyed, but also the other B complex vitamins, vitamins C, E, and beta carotene are as well. Furthermore, radioactive ions cause chromosomal damage and cell death in humans.

Irradiation is dangerous. People are led to believe that this process makes food safer. It creates, it is claimed, food which is seemingly microbe-free. Yet, when ingested, it damages all the organs in the body. This is through damage to genetic material. It isn't even required by law to label irradiated food. So, there is no way to avoid buying such disgusting material. This makes organic food a better buy and a safer choice. Also, even a patio or window garden can produce fresh dynamic food, and this saves on the grocery bill. The kits for growing hydroponic-type plants with pills that are added to water may not be adequate nutritionally. Furthermore, they do not contain heirloom seeds. Yet, this system seems to grow plants prolifically. It is possible to replace the seeds with the heirloom varieties and add liquid minerals and vitamins to the water. Thus, this would be an excellent way to grow natural food for consumption at home. Children (all people) must have safe and healthy food.

How riboflavin functions in the body

Just as thiamine works its magic on carbohydrates, riboflavin is also necessary to help change sugars and starches into energy. Combined with protein and phosphoric acid, enzymes are formed for the breakdown of blood sugar which is converted into energy. Five or more enzyme systems require riboflavin, and these actions affect amino acids, fatty acids, and carbohydrates. It also helps the cells to maintain the appropriate oxygen levels by supporting oxygen metabolism in the mitochondria (the lungs of a cell). This nutrient is absolutely essential just to maintain life.

When laboratory animals were deprived of riboflavin, they did not survive. Even when mildly deficient, their growth was slowed or stopped depending on the severity. The riboflavin deficient females frequently gave birth to deformed babies.

Everyone must eat riboflavin-rich foods daily, since supplementation with the synthetic form in vitamin pills is questionable. Also, many riboflavin supplements are made through genetic engineering. Children are frequently deficient in riboflavin. Because it is so easily destroyed by light and food processing, adequate natural sources are difficult to find. For riboflavin-rich wild, raw greens extracts see www.Americanwildfoods.com.

Deficiency symptoms and illnesses

When riboflavin is deficient, there is inflammation and tissue breakdown. Wounds fail to heal and, in fact, may become rapidly inflamed. Kids who heal slowly are, no doubt, riboflavin deficient.

When there is soreness plus cracks, scaling, and softening at the corners of the mouth, those are major deficiency signs. I have even had to inform health professionals that they were suffering from these symptoms, which are known as stomatitis. A particularly difficult case was solved simply by adding unsweetened, organic, full-fat yogurt to the diet. There may also be cracks and irritation around the nose, when the deficiency is severe enough.

Not only are the corners of the mouth affected, but also the lips and tongue. The lips may turn red, feel dry and burn, and easily crack open (cheilosis). Always check your child's tongue, just like good doctors do. If it is red, appears swollen, fissured, or inflamed, ask your child if his/her tongue feels like it is burning or if there is a problem with swallowing. If any or all of these symptoms are apparent, there is definitely a riboflavin deficiency. This important vitamin may even be almost nonexistent.

If a somewhat greasy scaling around the edges of the scalp occurs, this is called seborrheic dermatitis. No matter how often the hair is washed with the best organic shampoos and conditioners, it just doesn't go away. By increasing riboflavin immediately, it will simply disappear along with any pimples and flushing of the face. Yes, riboflavin is beneficial for those with chronic skin problems such as acne. For best results this important B vitamin found in wholesome food must be consumed on a daily basis.

Nervous symptoms can be quite irritating and even scary. These include numbness, burning feet, muscular weakness and difficulty walking, tremors, shaking, mental apathy, and dizziness. Sometimes these symptoms are even confused with diseases like MS and other neuromuscular diseases. Children are not exempt from the effects of vitamin deficiency and are actually more susceptible than adults because of their developmental requirements.

As a child around nine years of age I suffered from a severe riboflavin deficiency. My eyelids became severely scaly and sore as a result of a typical American diet full of sugar, white flour, commercial sweetened cereals, and little that was truly nourishing. It was a condition called granulated eyelids, and sties were also a frequent painful nuisance. My concerned parents took me to an ophthalmologist. He cauterized my eyelids with a hot needle. Not only did it scare me half to death, but it was also very painful. He had not even a clue that it was due to a vitamin deficiency. The painful and ugly condition wasn't resolved until I began sneaking the little packages of yeast out of the refrigerator and eating them—just because for some reason they tasted so good. They were intended for the big fluffy loaves of white bread that Mother made. She couldn't imagine what happened to the yeast. It wasn't until years later that I realized the riboflavin in the yeast was the miracle cure for those sore eyes.

Other eye complaints due to this vitamin deficiency include sensitivity to light, watering, blurry vision, dimness of sight, burning of the eyes, twilight blindness, conjunctivitis, disorders of the cornea, inflamed iris, inflamed optic nerve, gritty sensation of the eyelids, and dilation of the pupils. These eye problems are rarely associated with nutritional deficiency. Yet, B_2 deficiency is the most likely cause rather than a "deficiency" of antibiotics or some other form of medicine, which is commonly prescribed. B_2 or riboflavin works with vitamin A to prevent or eliminate these symptoms. These vitamins should be prescribed as the treatment of choice. Medications should be used only when all else fails due to secondary problems such as invasive infection. Natural food sources are always preferable, but severe symptoms may require aggressive supplementation. There are natural food source supplements for children, but they are difficult to find in most health food stores. These supplements plus yogurt added to a smoothie are an easy way to get the extra riboflavin. Organic egg yolk (soft boiled) will provide some riboflavin and vitamin A. Severe deficiency takes a considerable time to overcome, but using the natural food sources is the best way to relieve these chronic nutrition problems. Still, getting rid of the junk in children's diets is mandatory. Do not think that they are being deprived, because they are actually being rewarded with the resultant good health. The omitted candy bar will be long forgotten, but strength and good health throughout life is the greatest gift that a child can enjoy. Always keep in mind, whatever an individual thinks and believes is true—at least for him/her. If a person thinks and believes that he/she is always unlucky or deprived, then it is true. However, when the person reverses this negative thinking and begins to believe that he/she is blessed, then it is truly so.

Riboflavin sources and requirements

Riboflavin was first discovered in milk. It is also in yogurt. Do remember—when food is stored in clear glass containers and exposed to light, riboflavin is quickly destroyed. Real cheese—not fake cheese—may also be a good way to get a daily supply of riboflavin.

All food should be eaten as fresh as possible, since it quickly loses whatever valuable nutrients it contains. The majority of all food eaten should be fresh and uncooked—yes, raw. Of course, that means lots more vegetables. Other sources of riboflavin include leafy green vegetables and tomatoes, nutritional yeast, apricots, organic (only) lamb's or calf's liver and heart, organic beef, veal, buffalo, elk, and chicken. Do not eat chicken livers ever. They contain pathogens known to cause cancer. This was discovered by Dr. Virginia Livingston-Wheeler, the famous cancer researcher. Also, a natural, wild, raw liquid green food supplement is a good source of natural riboflavin. Children may take 5 drops to 1 dropperful daily, and the teen dosage is 2 to 3 droppersful daily. It is best absorbed under the tongue. However, for the fussy taster hide it in something such as tomato juice, grapefruit juice, soup, salad dressing, yogurt, honey—even mustard—whatever works to get it into the system.

Wouldn't it be great to have a tiny machine to pass over the food, and it would give a reading of the exact milligrams of all the nutrients within that food? That would certainly make life easier for everyone who is concerned with health. It would also provide a quick reference for all caring parents and guardians. None of us have any idea what nutrients we actually consume. That is what causes daily intake to be so controversial. However, if a recommended daily dose of a synthetic vitamin and mineral supplement is used and symptoms like those mentioned in this book are still occurring, there is a definite need for increasing the quantity of riboflavin (and other nutrients), which the child requires. A suggested minimal dosage for infants and small children is 1 to 4 mg, according to need, and this increases with age. Adults and teenagers require at a bare minimum 4 to 5 mg daily. However, with a high stress lifestyle and/or ill health children may need as much as 100 mg. A few examples of this may include those who have acne, diabetes, any digestive disorder, and cancer.

Many children and adults are riboflavin, as well as oxygen, deficient. While lecturing and doing body (symptom) readings all over the world, I have noticed that an increasing number of people of all ages are oxygen deprived. Certainly, the level of available oxygen in the air on this planet keeps decreasing, and riboflavin deficiency prevents cells from properly using whatever oxygen there is available to the body. With low oxygen in the tissues of the body, physical energy is affected and the risk of diseases such as hypothyroidism and cancer is increased, even in children. Research shows that there is a definite link between cancer and riboflavin deficiency. Cancer is an oxygen deficiency disease. When the cells are deprived of oxygen, cancer can and does grow prolifically. Certainly, the thyroid cannot work as it should when the body is oxygen starved. Just as a fire will not burn when there is no oxygen, the metabolism is adversely affected by a shortage of oxygen.

Many cancer patients have hypothyroidism. Chronically low body temperature is one of the many relevant signs of hypothyroidism. For an in-depth analysis and explanation of signs and symptoms of deficiencies and diseases and the significance of the body shape refer to the books *Nutrition Tests for Better Health* and *The Body Shape Diet,* by Dr. Cass Ingram. These signs are astoundingly accurate and more dependable than blood testing. This is because the body works very hard to maintain balance. It will take what is needed from the cells and make it available in the blood. Thus, the cells are affected first, and signs and symptoms frequently show up before the blood tests are abnormal. By the time the blood tests are abnormal, the body is damaged. Prevention with good nutrition is always the best medicine.

Niacin (B$_3$)

It was discovered in the 1930s that niacin had growth-stimulating properties and that it was an important substance in the heart. That is why children need niacin every day, and it is important for the strength of their physical structure for the remainder of their lives.

Niacin is present in every living cell. It plays a necessary part in the enzyme system in the body. Plus, it helps to promote the oxidative processes of the immune system for destruction of germs and for combustion of food. Furthermore, niacin aids in the transport of hydrogen atoms for the formation of hydrochloric acid. Thus, it is necessary for protein digestion and metabolism. It works together with riboflavin in cell metabolism, so symptoms of deficiency for both are quite similar. As with all B vitamins, niacin is vital for the human life force.

There are many conditions that are helped or relieved when niacin is increased on a daily basis. The following are some of the beneficial responses:

- relieves headaches
- relieves depression due to hypoglycemia
- helps eliminate symptoms of sugar withdrawal
- may help increase energy level
- may improve or help control appetite
- helps control/eliminate canker sores
- helps eliminate bad breath
- large doses may help schizophrenic behavior
- helps with leg cramps
- improves digestion/relieves indigestion
- provides protection from tooth decay
- aids concentration

Pellagra: a niacin deficiency disease

Severe niacin deficiency results in a disease called pellagra (from pellagra meaning rough skin). It was first apparent in areas where corn was a staple food. Corn is deficient in tryptophan, an amino acid which is a precursor to niacin. Tryptophan is changed into niacin within the tissues rather than by action within the intestines. Therefore, if the diet is rich in tryptophan, niacin deficiency is unlikely. Also, in the 1800s it was determined that pellagra was common among people who ate no flesh foods or cheese. They were obviously deficient in the amino acid, tryptophan commonly found in those foods.

Pellagra is always known in textbooks for its four "d's:" dermatitis, diarrhea, dementia, and death. Thus, it affects the skin, intestinal tract, and nerves. People are suffering from various stages of subclinical pellagra even today. One of the early signs is a red sore tongue. Other signs include fatigue without cause, fear without a reason, depression, and an inability to sleep. It is usually not recognized as a deficiency disease, and it is regularly treated with medications. Pasteur and others developed the germ theory for disease in the late 1800s. Unfortunately, modern medicine is still stuck in that realm, and many cases of outright nutritional deficiency are never diagnosed. Therefore, without a proper diagnosis, any treatment provided is most likely inappropriate.

The liver is the main storage area for niacin. With liver disease niacin may not be stored or properly used. Protein deficiency is a major cause of liver damage and niacin depletion. A steady diet of limited food choices low in protein, such as cereals, corn, corn syrup, rice, oats, certain fruits and vegetables, such as sweet potatoes and yams, will eventually result in symptoms of niacin deficiency or perhaps even pellagra. This means that the vegan diet especially is too limited. Vegetarians who eat eggs and cheeses are less likely to be deficient, but any meat-free diet should be supplemented. Certain types of torula yeast contain as much as 60% protein, plus all of the B vitamins, and much more. This yeast must be appropriately prepared as food. The wrong forms of yeast can actually grow inside the body and are harmful rather than helpful.

Deficiency symptoms and illnesses

One of the first symptoms of niacin deficiency is the very tip of the tongue is red, and further back it is covered with a white coating. In severe cases the coating on the tongue is black. Even animals can have black tongues due to nutritional deficiency, when they have a steady diet of poor quality pet food laced with corn. In Chinese natural medicine when the tip of the tongue is red, it means that there is a heart abnormality. This is definitely related to niacin depletion. Bad breath is also common, along with a furred tongue. Then, canker sores in the mouth often erupt, indicating a need for niacin. Almost always these sores are due to allergic reactions as well.

Stomach trouble and poor digestion result from lack of niacin. Hydrochloric acid may be low or non-existent due to the lack of niacin for hydrogen ion transport. With low or no hydrochloric acid more troubles are sure to result, since it is needed for the assimilation of protein, iron, and calcium. Vertical ridges on the fingernails indicate a deficiency in protein, iron, and calcium. Anemia, nerve disorders, poor bone integrity, and failure to thrive may be the ultimate result. Once it was rare to see ridged nails among children, but now all of the symptoms and signs mentioned are becoming more common. Each generation increasingly shows more signs of weakening due to poor diet and high stress lifestyles.

When the digestion is malfunctioning, many symptoms arise. Food is not broken down and absorption is impaired. Then, there is gas, bloating, constipation, or diarrhea. As time goes by the intestinal tract becomes increasingly inflamed with the rectum and anus most affected. Then colitis may develop. By the time the child reaches the teen years, so much inflammation is established that this activates additional problems such as anorexia, hormonal imbalances, acne, and more.

Other common signs of niacin deficiency are frequently experienced by children and adults as well. These signs include:

- dizziness
- irritability
- vomiting
- feeling of strain/tension
- crying or feel like crying
- sugar craving
- dark, scaly dermatitis
- nausea
- insomnia
- frequent headaches
- deep depression
- inability to concentrate
- weakness/lassitude
- disoriented/confused

Many of these symptoms are associated with the difficult child. An immediate behavior change may occur with the administration of a good natural supplement containing niacin plus protein-rich food. Tryptophan-rich foods are important, because trytophan may be converted into niacin, if needed. Sesame and tahini are rich in trytophan as are turkey, chicken, pheasant, beef, mackerel, and cottage cheese.

Niacin sources and requirements

The richest sources of niacin are wheat germ, yeast, liver, meat, and fish. Other good sources are eggs, nuts, dairy, mushrooms, legumes, tomato sauce, chunky peanut butter, avocado, baked potato, and wheat bran. All of these foods are best when they are from organic sources, which are unadulterated with chemicals and additives. Foods rich in tryptophan, such as turkey, sesame seed/tahini, milk, and yogurt, are always good choices, since this amino acid is converted to niacin.

To be able to function, the minimal daily dose for children is 4 to 15 mg according to the age of the child. For teens and adults the minimal daily dose is 20 to 30 mg. Frequently, a much larger amount is required, especially when the deficiency state has been prolonged, and there are many deficiency symptoms. A large intake of niacin (250 to 500 mg) may cause a severe flushing of the skin especially on the face. That is why focusing on food sources is much better, but it is difficult to obtain enough in food to be therapeutic. The niacin in all so-called fortified food is synthetic. A natural form of niacin supplement is from rice bran/polish drink mixes. The berry shake recipe on page 98 is a delightful way to nourish the whole family. There is also a potent natural B complex powder high in niacin. Made from torula yeast, rice bran, and royal jelly it is the most dense natural source of niacin known.

While good organic or wild food is the best medicine, it is often mentioned that normal healthy food may disrupt the activity of medication. However, keep in mind that niacin is compromised by taking drugs such as antibiotics. Actual deficiency can be produced when taking such medications.

Hopefully, there would never be any long term use of such drugs, but niacin supplementation is a must for those who continuously take them.

Niacin is not readily destroyed when exposed to the air or heat. However, it is lost in water during cooking. Since it is water soluble, prolonged soaking of food is discouraged. Thus, beans, legumes, and peas may lose some of the little niacin that they contain when the soaking water is discarded. However, nuts and seeds soaked overnight absorb the water, begin to sprout, and provide even higher amounts of vitamins than the usual type.

Many children and especially teenagers are severely deficient in this vitamin. Under those conditions it may be impossible to replenish their bodies with sufficient niacin solely through the diet. Thus, supplements may be needed, and megadoses may be required. It is wise to use a natural B vitamin supplement which contains all the B vitamins and co-factors. The purely natural B complex powder is one such supplement. Improvements in behavior and overall health are noticed within a week or so, but daily supplementation is usually required for at least six months or longer. Thereafter, a daily maintenance dose is beneficial.

Pantothenic acid (B₅)

Pantothenic acid is found in almost every living being. It is within the tissues throughout the body. That means it is vital for energy and life. It is especially important for the adrenal glands, which are the coping mechanisms of the body. They help kids, as well as moms and dads, remain calm, cool, and collected. That is what everyone wants and needs most of all.

How pantothenic acid (B₅) functions in the body

The intestines make a certain amount of pantothenic acid from intestinal bacteria. Like the other B vitamins its main function is as a coenzyme in the metabolism of carbohydrates, fatty acids, and amino acids. It even plays a role in the production of cholesterol, adrenal steroid hormones, and the sex hormones. Pantothenic acid is involved in the first step of the formation of hemoglobin, the oxygen-carrying substance in the red blood cells.

In a research study rats deprived of pantothenic acid had coarse scant hair. The hair coat is always an indicator of health, even in humans. During the study the rats failed to grow and develop. Plus, their blood, lungs, and stomachs were damaged. In the blood the antibodies and phagocytes were reduced. That means the immune system was injured. While rats are certainly different than humans, the results of the study are important. It helps to pinpoint similar damage commonly found in humans. Since children are growing and developing, they are far more sensitive to diets deprived of important nutrients. These deficiency symptoms are very evident in their physical development and emotional behavior.

Deficiency symptoms and illnesses

Since pantothenic acid is important in so many functions in the body, no one can afford to be deficient in this vitamin. It works as a coenzyme with the other B vitamins in the breakdown of nutrients and in the formation of natural steroids. When it is deficient, the adrenals are severely damaged. The adrenals make over sixty hormones. While the amounts of the hormones needed are tiny, they are vital for normal functioning of the body. They work kind of like Christmas tree lights. When a light is burned out, the rest of the lights will not work either. Hormones activate or generate an action in the body, and they must be available for all systems to work correctly.

Some children complain about burning on the soles of their feet as do many adults. Not only is this painful, but it makes walking difficult. In the Orient in labor camps during World War II the American prisoners suffered excruciating pain from burning feet. When they were treated with pantothenic acid, the pain was relieved.

The tongue is always a good indicator for B vitamin deficiency, and pantothenic acid is no exception. When the tongue appears large, beefy, and furrowed and the individual suffers from eczema, this is a common sign of pantothenic acid deficiency.

Pantothenic acid sources and requirements

As with most B vitamins yeast, liver and kidney are the best sources for pantothenic acid. Other acceptable sources are egg yolk and skimmed milk. Skimmed milk contains more than whole milk due to the higher water content. Even so, whole milk is better for drinking. A milk sugar called galactose causes gastric irritation and even cancer could develop over a period of time, when there is no fat present to protect the tissue. Fair sources are lean beef, whole milk, cheese, broccoli, kale, sweet potatoes, yellow corn, and legumes. Organic food contains higher quantities than the commercial types.

Since pantothenic acid is a water soluble vitamin, it is lost in the urine and perspiration. If the adrenal glands are weak and the individual is under a lot of stress, the need for this vitamin increases. Frequent urination indicates adrenal stress. Direly, it could also be a sign of diabetes. Therefore, if this symptom occurs, additional pantothenic acid is needed. A children's formula of raw royal jelly pudding-like mixture is a good supplemental source of this vital nutrient, as is the purely natural B complex powder.

Resources differ, but children require a minimum of 1 to 5 mg daily depending on age, size, weight, activity, stress and adrenal integrity. Hot climates and severely cold climates also create a greater need for children and adults alike. Adults lose around 3 to 10 mg daily, so a minimal intake should be no less that 20 mg daily. Many children and adults require more than this. Even just an adequate amount of this nutrient increases physical and mental tolerance. If a child is hyperactive and disagreeable, this vitamin may well be the answer to curbing or even eliminating such symptoms. No doubt, adrenal support is beneficial.

Pyridoxine (B$_6$)

When research animals developed a certain form of dermatitis, Szent Gyorgyi isolated pyridoxine as the missing necessary substance. Infants and young children with pink disease also exhibited B$_6$ deficiency, as do children with mercury intoxication from vaccinations with thimerasol. The symptoms of B$_6$ deficiency are troublesome and can be quite severe or even deadly. They include edema, skin rash, excessively pink-colored arms and legs with scarlet cheeks and nose, heavy sweating, digestive disturbances, sensitivity to light, nerve damage, periods of extreme irritability, alternating with listlessness and apathy, inflammatory changes in the central nervous system, and failure to thrive.

Mercury, a highly dangerous substance, destroys pyridoxine and poisons the child. Vaccinations should be refused. Doctors in England recently stated that babies should not have vaccinations due to their toxicity. Further, they noted that the vaccines have no value, since the babies' immune systems are not yet established. The physical health and intelligence of a child are at risk. (See Appendix B, pages 321-324 for a religious exemption form.) Some doctors will work with parents to avoid vaccinations. The perils of vaccinations are revealed by Dr. Tenpenny's *Saying No To Vaccines* and Dr. Ingram's *The Cause for Cancer Revealed*.)

How pyridoxine (B$_6$) functions in the body

Pyridoxine's main function is to help the body utilize proteins and fats. Its role in brain chemistry is crucial. This vitamin regulates the neurons. Brain activity is affected by the conversion of glutamic acid and tryptophan, two important amino acids. This conversion is dependent on B$_6$. The production of energy is also a significant function of this vitamin. Additionally, it is involved in the production of hemoglobin, the oxygen-carrying compound in the blood. Plus, B$_6$ is required for the transport of amino acids across the intestinal wall.

Pyridoxine is actually a combination of compounds. As one of the compounds of pyridoxine, pyridoxal phosphate is active as a co-enzyme. This means without pyridoxine there would be no growth, the brain would not function appropriately, the amino acid metabolism would be impeded, and the transport of nutrients into the cells would be inhibited.

It is possible to take too much of this vitamin, but only when the dosages are massive and for a prolonged period. Fortunately, the neurological symptoms are resolved when supplementation is stopped. Even so, it is virtually impossible to overdose on food sources. For best absorption and function in the body magnesium must also be available. B_6 and magnesium are the great energizers and can quickly restore physical energy and mental well-being. Therefore, if a child appears to be listless, flaccid, and lazy, he/she could well be missing this important B vitamin and mineral combination.

Deficiency symptoms and illnesses

Hardening of the arteries is thought to occur only in the elderly. However, autopsies were done on eighteen year old boys killed in World War II, and even they had clogged arteries. Children are not immune from such conditions, when their diets are deficient. Every day a mother fed her toddler hard teething biscuits made from white flour, along with bologna, occasionally a few overcooked vegetables, and pasteurized cow's milk. He became obese and cranky. When tested, his cholesterol was very high. The doctors placed him on a very strict calorie-restricted diet. He did lose weight, and his cholesterol was reduced. Just getting him off the nitrate-loaded, sugar-infested bologna was an improvement. However, what he really needed was a good wholesome fresh food diet high in the vital nutrients. Today, he is a big, strong-looking, young man with a weak heart.

Dr. Schroeder of the Department of Internal Medicine at Washington University School of Medicine in St. Louis confirmed that pyridoxine deficiency in the diet of experimental monkeys resulted in hardening of the arteries.

When a similar experiment was done with rats, it caused high blood pressure. These same animals suffered with decreased antibody formation/immune function (low white blood cells) and increased susceptibility to infection. They readily developed pneumonia and other infections. Further symptoms continued to occur due to B_6 deficiency. The laboratory animals developed skin lesions, anemia, cardiovascular disease, fatty degeneration of the liver, kidney disease, and nerve lesions. When infants were fed a faulty formula deficient in B_6, they became highly irritable and ultimately suffered from convulsions. Most importantly, the seizures stopped when B_6 was added to the formula.

It should come as no surprise that according to the book *The Vitamins in Medicine,* by Bicknell and Prescott, vitamin B_6 has been used clinically for the tough cases of neuromuscular illnesses. Those with muscular dystrophy, Parkinson's disease, multiple sclerosis, carpal tunnel syndrome, and other serious diseases have benefited greatly from using pyridoxine as a supplement. Other deficiency symptoms, including tremors and nervous tics, improved with this vitamin treatment. It also acts as an effective diuretic. Pregnant women suffering from severe nausea and vomiting respond well to supplementation. Radiation victims also benefited from additional B_6. With all the exposure to radiation at airports now, it is advisable to make sure the whole family has adequate vitamin B_6 intake and an additional boost when flying. Also with depleted uranium arriving on the winds and contaminating the air, the food chain, the earth, and all water sources, B_6 deficiency is a greater danger than ever before.

Many of the diseases mentioned were at one time common only among the aged. That was mostly due to impaired digestion as people grew older, and they ate less food or a less healthy diet. Now with normal food sources so depleted, even children are suffering from the so-called diseases of the elderly. To meet even minimal requirements, supplementation/food fortification is needed on a daily basis. Good natural whole food sources include torula and brewer's yeast, undiluted raw high-grade royal jelly, and crude whole rice fractions, which contain the germ and the bran.

Pyridoxine (B₆) sources and requirements

Most of the foods that contain the other B vitamins also contain B_6. Many foods contain very small amounts, but good sources are from torula or brewer's yeast, brown rice, wild rice, wheat germ and bran, corn, peas, beans, lentils, peanuts, liver, kidney, various meats, and fish. Smaller amounts are found in milk, egg yolk, pecans, green leafy vegetables, cabbage, and cantaloupe.

Daily intake for all humans should never fall below 2 to 4 mg. Ideally, the amount should be considerably more, around 50 mg daily for children over 5 years. Pyridoxine is considered to be quite harmless, and usually it is obviously deficient in those who regularly consume processed/refined foods from the grocery store. However, it may be produced by bacterial synthesis in the intestines. Just how much would be synthesized is unknown, and the amount would vary according to the health status of the individual.

Vitamin B₁₂

This vitamin was discovered as a result of the search for a cure for pernicious anemia. It was found that liver and liver concentrates were curative, and finally it was isolated into a crystalline form. Cobalt was the essential component in the molecule. It was named B_{12} and also called cyanocobalamine. Other forms today are methylcobalamine and hydroxycobalamine with the latter being the best form to use for supplementation.

There are several factors which inhibit B_{12} absorption, and the result is anemia. For absorption to occur the stomach must produce a substance known as intrinsic factor as well as hydrochloric acid. A shortage of calcium and the intake of laxatives, which force the food through the intestines before absorption is completed, are also factors which retard the body's absorption of this vitamin. Also, antacids and H-2 blockers disrupt stomach acid secretions and, therefore, lead to deficiency. This is very important for pregnant women and nursing mothers. It seems there is a relationship between B_{12} deficiency and the development of mongoloidism.

Disease and B_{12}

Pernicious anemia causes nerve cell damage in the spinal cord. The results of this damage are a jerky manner of walking, swaying, lack of coordination, and loss of balance. B_{12} is needed for nerve cell repair, and without it cells die. It is also needed in the formation of red blood cells, and along with folic acid it will eliminate pernicious anemia.

These are other diseases that respond to B_{12}.

- ulcers
- rheumatoid arthritis
- muscular dystrophy
- psoriasis
- bursitis
- migraines
- shingles
- hepatitis

- asthma
- osteoporosis
- sciatica
- osteoarthritis
- sprue/celiac disease
- multiple sclerosis

B_{12} is rarely found in plants except for maca, chaga, chlorella, and spirulina. The B_{12} in maca and chaga is absorbed, but from algae it is questionable. Thus, vegans have limited amounts, if any, of this vitamin from food. Fine sources of raw royal jelly may provide a trace of B_{12}. The two new vegetable sources which may help are raw purple maca and raw chaga extract. The extracts are taken as drops under the tongue. These examples are natural food sources as opposed to synthetic derivatives.

B_{12} sources and requirements

The best food sources of vitamin B_{12} are liver and kidney. Meat, milk, cheese, eggs, royal jelly, torula yeast, and fish are fair sources. Fruits, vegetables, seeds and nuts do not contain this vitamin. Algae, maca, and chaga mushroom are the only other potential sources.

As with all vitamins the requirement varies with individual need. Daily intake from food is best, and the minimal recommendation is around 2 to 10 micrograms. Infants and children require 2 micrograms or more, while teenagers require around 10 micrograms. During illness the requirement increases. Vegans may require injections of B_{12} and folic acid to maintain health and strength. The importance of this nutrient cannot be ignored or neglected. Over time the symptoms become more evident, and they are mostly irreversible. Since the American diet is so inadequate, more and more people are affected.

How B_{12} helps nerves, the brain, and body functions

B_{12} is essential for maintaining the myelin sheath around the nerves. It is much like the covering around electric wires. If this breaks down, the nerves are short-circuited and damaged. The myelin is composed of fatty acids, which B_{12} directly controls. Thus, nerve damage is certain when B_{12} is depleted. The nerves control every movement of the body, and they affect coping skills and mental stability.

In B_{12} deficiency the brain suffers damage. Apathy, moodiness, poor memory, fearfulness, and confusion are certain signs of lack of B_{12}. So is depression.

Muscle fatigue, low energy, and poor appetite are often a problem for children of all ages and throughout the teen years. This especially is true for girls who are weight watching or even anorexic. Because of poor food choices and low caloric food intake B_{12} is often a missing component in their daily diets. Even if the teen consumes massive calories, the sources of B_{12} are limited and are not likely to be common choices or favorite food selections among the teen population.

Folic acid and B_{12} are a team. B_{12} actually supports the appropriate function of folic acid in the body. Both help support the immune system against infection, especially in newborn babies. B_{12} provides a sense of well-being and energy. It, along with folic acid, is truly an important vitamin for growing, learning, and thriving children.

Note: A vegan diet is not recommended for children. Recently, in New York a toddler died from starvation and failure to thrive on a vegan diet, which means no meat, milk or eggs. No doubt the parents were following their belief system and meant no harm to the child. However, both parents were imprisoned due to the death of the child. In another case strict vegans fed the child only vegetable matter, and the mother during pregnancy only ate vegetation. Thus, the child was deficient in certain nutrients, such as B_{12} and B_2, and is a mongoloid. When a child fails to grow and develop, it is necessary to find the reason and resolve it. Children need more nutrients, because they are forming their skeletal systems, immune systems, and physical status for the rest of their lives. Without the proper nutrients this cannot be achieved.

Infection of the gut can lead to deficiency. For example, a thirteen-year-old boy in England went on a holiday with his parents to Sudan. The boy ate food from street vendors. He became quite ill, and his family quickly returned to London.

After many tests and three months in the hospital, it was determined that he had aplastic anemia from parasites picked up from the street food. Parasite infections are more common than most people think. B_{12} deficiency can occur whenever the gut is disturbed to such a degree. Aplastic anemia, as well as other types of anemia, is life threatening. B_{12} deficiency is the cause of several forms of anemia.

Folic Acid

Folic acid compounds were discovered in 1941 by the research team Mitchell, Snell, and Williams. It was found to be most prolific in spinach and liver.

Folic acid and B_{12} *both* are important in the prevention of anemia. B_{12} is needed for the full recovery of patients with pernicious anemia, and folic acid will prevent macrocytic anemia of pregnancy and megaloblastic anemia of infancy. When the mother is treated and cured with folic acid, the nursing baby will appropriately respond to the folic acid from the mother's milk. It is presumed that the beneficial effects of folic acid would mask the need for B_{12}, which is the actual cure for pernicious anemia. Therefore, folic acid supplements have been limited to 400 mcg per serving. This makes it difficult to take larger doses even when the need and the deficiency exist. For best results folic acid and B_{12} should be taken together when administered as a supplement or as an injection.

How folic acid functions in the body

It is now proven that a deficiency of folic acid is the cause of birth defects such as spina bifida. Folic acid is necessary for normal division of living cells. That is why all men and women of childbearing age must be certain to have enough folic acid before pregnancy. Hangnails indicate such a deficiency and are an easy, yet important clue that the body needs folic acid. This also means that the digestive system is in trouble, since the cells that line the gut are the fastest to renew—about every six days. If folic acid is lacking, the digestive system fails to regenerate. Thus, digestion and absorption of vital nutrients are impaired. Sprue (celiac disease) is a gastrointestinal disease, which responds to folic acid treatment. It is becoming increasingly common. The symptoms include internal lesions, malabsorption and poor nutritional status, diarrhea, and macrocytic anemia. Folic acid is the treatment of choice for this serious condition and the resolution of the many symptoms.

The ultimate function of folic acid and B_{12} seems to be in bringing the blood into contact with all the tissues. Also, it facilitates cell growth, blood-forming factors, and even DNA. If that doesn't get you to eat spinach and those dark green veggies, nothing will. Remember, it is good for the blood and—Popeye would agree—it supplies powerful energy.

Deficiency symptoms and illnesses

Again, one of the first clues of folic acid deficiency is hangnails. However, glossitis (inflammation of the tongue) and diarrhea may be present and are actually quite common. Anemia, gastrointestinal disorders, low (or lack of) hydrochloric acid in the stomach, and low white blood cell count are a result of insufficient folic acid. Celiac disease, a chronic intestinal disorder in infants and children, responds well and fairly quickly to treatment with folic acid. The problem is only nutritionally aware doctors are familiar with this treatment—the only really appropriate one.

Folic acid sources and requirements

Children who are deficient respond rapidly to fresh food sources of folic acid. Today, kids have such sweet cravings that they find vegetables unappealing. However, fresh raw veggie/fruit juice can be prepared quickly and easily with a home juice machine. Fresh is always best, so do not make a large amount and store it unless it is absolutely necessary. Folic acid is abundant in dark green leafy vegetables such as spinach and kale. The following juice is great for a daily supply of folic acid and much more.

Popeye's Punch (Folic Acid Blood Builder)

    1 cup fresh raw organic spinach carefully washed
    1 cup fresh raw organic kale carefully washed

1 quartered fresh organic apple (no seeds)
1 fresh organic orange, remove only the orange outer
   peel, leaving as much of the white as possible,
   because it contains important and inexpensive
   bioflavonoids. Cut into pieces.

Put ingredients into the juicer in the order listed. Blend and serve. Additionally, add one teaspoon of kid's formula royal jelly/pumpkinseed oil. Stir until dissolved. This makes the drink more nutrient dense. Royal jelly adds some B_{12}, which should be combined with folic acid. Also, one tablespoon of raw, wild honey or yacon syrup, a delicious natural sweetener from Peru high in inulin, can make this drink more tempting for those who crave sweets and sugar.

In both children and adults chronic sweet/sugar craving is a sure sign of fungal overgrowth in the body. For a complete explanation of fungal problems and how to cope with them, read Dr. Cass Ingram's book, *The Cure is in the Cupboard.*

Other sources of folic acid are from organic liver and kidney, but these are rarely eaten today. If you do decide to add these nutritious organ meats to your menu, you MUST use ONLY organic. Even the animals are toxic today from being fed genetically modified grain and ground up animal refuse made into innocent-looking feed pellets. Animals should only consume their natural forage and organic feed. More people are eating less and less meat and for good reason. If you don't eat meat, then organic milk, eggs, cheese, and royal jelly are a must, especially for growing children.

For those who are deficient in folic acid and B_{12} and have significant symptoms, there is an absolutely delicious paté that can be made from organic lamb's or calf's liver that most kids can be enticed to eat on bread, crackers, or fresh celery or carrot sticks.

Perfect Paté

- ½ pound lamb's liver or calf's liver cut into small pieces, use ONLY organic
- 1 small onion or two green onions, chopped (optional)
- 1 or more cloves of pressed garlic (optional)
- 3 tablespoons (about) olive oil or coconut/palm oil
- 8 sun-dried cherry tomato halves (in extra virgin olive oil)
- 1 carton (16 ounces) organic kefir cheese, quark (sour cream-like substances found only in health food or ethnic store), or sour cream
- 2 tablespoons capers
- 2 tablespoons chopped chives
- 4 to 6 pitted chopped olives
- 2 tablespoons finely chopped green pepper
- 2 tablespoons finely chopped red pepper
- 2 tablespoons finely chopped dill (optional)
- 1 teaspoon sea salt or garlic salt
- 1 tablespoon oregano spice mixture
- 1 tablespoon black seed spice mixture

In a small skillet sauté the liver, onion, and garlic in the extra virgin olive oil or coconut/palm oil, just until liver is slightly pink inside. Remove from heat and let cool. Drain any remaining oil and put the liver, onion, and garlic plus the sun-dried tomatoes into a blender. Blend on low speed until lightly puréed. In a large bowl combine the puréed liver, onions, garlic, and tomato with the kefir or quark, and add capers, chives, chopped olives, green pepper, red pepper, dill, sea salt or garlic salt, and the remaining herb and spice mixtures. Stir gently until all ingredients are mixed. Chill in the refrigerator, and spread on rice or whole grain crackers, rye or 7-grain bread as a sandwich, or use as a dip on organic chips and vegetable sticks. Even those who hate the taste of liver enjoy this paté, because the liver taste is virtually gone. If there are ingredients that you do not like (other than the liver), leave them out. If you leave out the liver, it makes a great dip, but the liver is the source of folic acid and B_{12}.

For those who do not want to cut and chop, just put all ingredients in the blender with the liver, onions, and garlic and blend until smooth. It will have a different color, taste, and texture, but it is still delicious. It takes less time and is almost as tasty and just as nutritious.

Like riboflavin, light destroys folic acid and so does high or excessive heat during cooking. Fresh, dark green salads are great vitamin sources. Kids can help wash the leaves to remove grit, sand, contaminants, and even parasites. Even the prewashed salad greens should be rinsed in clean water. (People pick up parasites from unwashed produce.) Teach kids to gently tear the leaves into bite-sized pieces—do not cut up the greens with a knife. Do not use iceberg lettuce, since it contains little nourishment. Chopped cherry tomatoes and carrots and sprouts carefully washed are a perfect addition. Vegans should use avocado in salad to balance blood sugar and for more nourishment. Almonds, sunflower seeds, sesame seeds, flax seeds, pumpkin seeds, and other nuts and seeds can be covered in clean water and soaked over night. Then, drain any remaining water, and add the nut and seed combination to the salad. This makes the nuts and seeds easier to chew and digestion is more complete—thus, they are far more nourishing. Sun chokes, which are also called Jerusalem artichokes, are rich in a substance called inulin. This helps stabilize blood sugar and helps to quell the infernal sugar craving. Other vegetables which are tasty and truly beneficial are capers (especially beneficial for the liver), artichoke hearts packed in water—not oil unless it is extra virgin olive oil, hearts of palm, turnips, parsley and parsley root, radishes, mushrooms if tolerated, raw sweet potato, chopped onion and garlic (a bit strong for some children, but can be lightly sautéed in coconut/palm oil and then added to food), shredded, raw or cooked beets and greens, green beans and so on. Soup is also wonderful, easy, and nourishing. Just use the "stone soup" method: dump in what you like. First, sauté the onions and garlic in a little extra virgin olive oil or coconut/palm oil until softened.

Note: A soup bone or stew meat can be added at this time with the onions and garlic, and when the meat and onions and garlic are lightly browned add about 6 to 8 cups of water. Use medium heat and cook the bone for broth and stew meat until tender for at least two hours or more. Then, remove from the heat and take out the bone. Let the broth cool and skim any fat off the top of the broth. An easier method is to cool the broth overnight in the refrigerator. The fat will harden and float on top of the broth. This makes it easy to remove excess fat. Then, add more water, tomato juice, or vegetable juice if needed to the stock and any vegetables desired such as chopped carrots, potatoes, green beans, celery, cabbage, peppers, and tomatoes and cook just until the vegetables are tender. Season to taste with sea salt, pepper, and 1 heaping teaspoon of the oregano spice mixture, plus 4 or more vegetable bouillon cubes.

For a vegetarian soup add to the sautéed onions and garlic 4 to 6 cups of water, potatoes with skin (no green should show under the skin ever, since this is caused by a poisonous substance called solanine, which develops when potatoes are exposed to light), carrots, green beans or other beans, beets, broccoli, cauliflower, Jerusalem artichoke, or any other vegetable you have available fresh or left over plus sea salt and herbal seasonings such as 1 or 2 teaspoons of oregano spice mixture and/or 1 or 2 teaspoons of herbal/fenugreek spice mixture and/or black seed spice mixture. Cook just until vegetables are tender. If more liquid is needed you may wish to add 1 or 2 cups of tomato or vegetable juice to taste for additional flavor and nourishment. Conventional non-organic juices most likely contain GMO contamination. I add fresh raw organic vegetable juice at the end of the cooking time. Use your imagination and try new and unusual foods. I make uncooked soup in the Vita Mix. Merely use any fresh vegetables normally used in soups, 2 to 4 tablespoons of pure cold-pressed sesame or pumpkinseed oil, and sea salt/seasonings that you enjoy, blend until pureed, and immediately add 2 to 3 cups of boiling water. This instant soup is so delicious that it is hard to eat cooked soup after you try this. Parents can't be picky and expect any better behavior from the kids. Try new things. Get excited about new ways to eat better, and the kids will pick up on this positive approach to growing more healthy.

With all those wonderful vegetables the dressing should be just as exciting and nourishing. Austrian cold-pressed pumpkinseed oil, pure cold-pressed sesame and black seed oil, along with pure apple cider vinegar, rice vinegar, or a good balsamic vinegar are excellent for dressings. Just pour over salad or chopped/shredded vegetables and eat. However, do not forget to eat the dressing and encourage the kids to do so. Why? The dressing aids digestion and is also protective against bacteria and other contaminants which are, hopefully, never present. These dressing ingredients contain the important essential fatty acids, vitamins, and minerals, and it aids digestive processes for those with low stomach acid. Kids might not like it at first, but if they see you or other children eating it, they will too. The following recipe is easy, tasty, and full of the best health giving nutrients.

Green Dragon Dressing

¼ cup Austrian cold-pressed pumpkinseed oil
¼ cup cold-pressed sesame oil
2 tablespoons cold-pressed black seed oil
¼ cup extra virgin olive oil
¾ cup vinegar—raw apple cider, rice vinegar, or Balsamic (if vinegar is too strong use ½ cup vinegar and ¼ cup veggie broth or tomato juice)
2 tablespoons mustard
1 teaspoon sea salt or garlic salt
1 tablespoon oregano spice mixture
1 tablespoon paprika
1 tablespoon raw wild honey (optional)
   Dried chopped dill, parsley, thyme, and rosemary

(optional) that you make yourself or buy organic brands only—others are irradiated. 1 teaspoon of each or more if desired.

Combine all ingredients in a blender and blend until thoroughly mixed. Chill in the refrigerator, and shake well before serving over salad and vegetables.

Children need a bare minimum of around 2 to 4 mg daily of folic acid for growth and tissue repair. Teens require 5 to 10 mg daily. When a deficiency disease is present, a much higher requirement would be indicated. Again, folic acid supplementation is always best with B_{12}. Unfortunately, only 400 mcg tablets or capsules are available. Doctors can prescribe 1 mg tablets. Yet, food sources are far superior, and you are spending your hard earned dollars on food to fill and furnish the body with what it needs to grow, develop, and repair. Wild and organic foods, as well as real food supplements, nourish children with what they need, not just synthetic, sugar sweetened, chemicals called multiple vitamins. Save your money for real food, and do your children a favor by helping their bodies to vigorously grow and be strong and healthy for a lifetime.

B vitamin co-factors

This all sounds pretty complex, but if you have an understanding of why something works or doesn't work, everything gets easier. It is no fun for you or your child to experience ill health, fatigue, poor digestion, constipation, diarrhea, and all the symptoms and diseases that plague the human race. So let's continue through the co-factors, and what you learn will astound you. You don't have to remember it all. Just keep this book handy, underline the important parts which have a special meaning for you, and write notes, questions, and comments in the margins. Health professionals want to help, when there are troubling health issues. Yet, they may not have the understanding of nutrition in relation to the complexities of body chemistry and how important food is for growth and maintenance. It seems so obvious that food is fuel. When health issues arise, diet should be the first consideration. Unfortunately, it is usually last or never examined at all. What we don't know or understand, we do not pursue or admit any validity. Be informed or at least be aware that these facts exist, and know where to find them. Plus, keeping an open mind may be life saving for you and those you love.

PABA

PABA, inositol, choline, and biotin are also important components in the B complex vitamin family. PABA is actually a part of the folic acid molecule and the requirements, sources, and deficiency symptoms are basically the same as folic acid. PABA has been found to be beneficial for vitiligo, which appears as white spots or lack of pigment on the skin. This condition also indicates fungal infestation. It is also protective against sunburn damage, fatigue, anemia, and rashes. Drugs may block the beneficial enzyme reactions of this substance. The richest food sources are organic liver, molasses, brewer's and baker's yeast, royal jelly, and wheat germ. Basically, wherever there is an abundance of natural B vitamins, PABA is available too.

PABA is a better skin protective agent than sunscreen. Researchers at the University of Miami found that hairless mice, which were treated with PABA before being exposed to the damaging rays of UV light, were protected from the development of cancerous tumors. PABA protected their skin even when chemicals known to produce tumors under UV light were also used. UV rays only cause sunburn, and they do not tan the skin.

PABA is absorbed into the skin tissues. Thus, it is much more protective than the chemical lotions and creams that easily wash off when swimming and bathing. Also many of the chemical sunburn agents block too much of the sun's rays and that causes the skin to be unable to make vitamin D. This action has actually increased the incidence of skin cancers.

Research indicates that PABA is safe, and little to no known reaction is recorded. There is therapeutic evidence and research that PABA improves vitiligo conditions. This is important, because the light spots on the skin appear mostly where there is sun exposure. It also protects the skin from sunburn, plus it is essential in the production of body protein and synthesis of red blood cells. Daily intake of natural sources of this substance is important. Besides the organic food sources mentioned, torula yeast has become an important natural source of this necessary component in human nutrition.

Inositol

Inositol plays an important role in the growth process, and it is associated with choline and biotin. Mice given a diet deficient in inositol failed to grow, and they lost most all of their hair.

When they were fed inositol from yeast and liver, they regrew their hair within 18 days. Another rich source of inositol is from lecithin, but most all lecithin is from soy. Soy is mostly derived from genetically modified plants. If you use lecithin made from soy, be sure you have a written guarantee that it is not from genetically modified soy. Sunflower lecithin is a better choice, although difficult to obtain in the United States. To purchase this rare sunflower lecithin see www.Americanwildfoods.com. Other inositol sources are found in wheat germ, oatmeal, molasses, beans, peas, grapefruit, oranges, peaches, peanuts, potatoes, spinach, strawberries, tomatoes, and turnips.

Inositol is concentrated in muscles, the brain, red blood cells, the heart, and the kidneys. No doubt, children thrive and function better when their diets are rich in inositol and other B complex vitamins. There is a high concentration of inositol in the lens of the eye and in the muscles of the heart. Some children may need as much as 500 mg daily and teens around 1000 mg, since there is more inositol in the body than any other vitamin except for niacin.

Deficiency symptoms may be confused with other vitamins, because they are common for other nutrients too. Deficiency symptoms include constipation, eczema, and abnormalities of the eyes. Fortunately, this important nutrient is found in many fresh foods such as those mentioned earlier.

Choline

Like inositol, choline is a lipotropic agent. That means it is part of the process that keeps the body from developing a fatty liver. The liver is the most versatile and hardest working organ in the body besides the heart. When it fails to function, we are poisoned from the inside out, and we starve to death. The liver deals with all toxins and poisons, and it makes and/or stores glycogen, vitamin A, and other nutrients and enzymes. The liver also breaks down fats, carbohydrates, and proteins for the body's building material and nourishment of the cells. Thus, choline is a necessary factor for the body's handling of fats and cholesterol. High cholesterol can be reduced with choline supplementation. As mentioned before, even children can have occluded arteries. A well-rounded diet rich in the B complex vitamins helps to prevent this from happening, and these nutrients work together. For example, thiamine is necessary to prevent a choline deficiency.

The best natural sources are (sunflower seed) lecithin, wheat germ, liver, kidney, and eggs. It is so important that very little choline is excreted from the body, and yet, the requirement is fairly high. For children a minimum of 250 mg daily is required, and for teens a minimum of 650 mg is needed each day. The American junk food diet provides virtually none, and more and more people including children suffer liver damage and other dangerous conditions.

Biotin

Biotin is also important in the metabolism of fatty compounds, and it plays a role in growth and development. When you see children with "rooster tails" or hair that stands straight up at the back of the crown of the head, you can be sure they are biotin deficient. If you routinely put raw egg in food or drinks, such as smoothies, this can induce biotin deficiency. The raw egg white contains avidin, an enzyme which breaks down biotin. Yet, biotin is found in the yolk of the egg. Common deficiency symptoms are muscular pain, poor appetite, dry skin, nervous system disturbances, lack of energy and sleeplessness. So, your little night owl may be deficient in biotin, and the children's formula of royal jelly/pumpkinseed oil has lots.

Animals found to be deficient in biotin lost their fur especially around the eyes, had retarded growth, moved with a spastic walk, suffered from itchy dermatitis, developed heart and lung ailments, and were unable to reproduce and nurse. Puppies lacking in biotin developed a progressive paralysis.

Biotin is found in many of the same sources as choline and inositol. Yeast, liver, kidney, egg yolk, milk, peas, molasses, tomatoes, and unrefined cereals are good natural sources. Royal jelly is the top source of this vitamin. The requirement for children may be as high as 150 mg per day, and for teens 300 mg.

If children are raised on the Standard American Diet (it really is SAD), they will be deficient in the vital B complex vitamins and far more. This affects behavior, temperament, learning ability, and intelligence. It further affects growth and development. Loving and caring parents never wish to deprive their children and cause them to be less than what they are capable of being. However, are you at your wits end about why your child is always acting out or incapable of sleeping enough or sleeps too much? Does your child have little or no appetite or desires food non-stop and is gaining too much weight? Does he/she suffer from constant illnesses or allergies and is always negative and crying? Does your child have limited attention span? Is he/she nervous, agitated, moody, angry, and full of attitude? If so, help is desperately needed. Better food choices and eating habits, plus all the other good habits that go along with this, should be emphasized. Without change in diet and lifestyle he/she will suffer the consequences for the rest of his/her life.

As you read and digest this information, there may be symptoms that you have as well. It truly is time to make those changes as you begin to understand more and learn the secrets of good health. Keep pen and paper handy to write down ways that would be easy to introduce new and healthy changes into the household. Start today. Use trickery if you must such as secret recipes, which hide all the nutrient dense components. Stay away from uncooperative outsiders who belittle your efforts to change to a better way of life for your own immediate family circle. Know that you are on the right path, and ignore any ridicule. Just because everyone around is eating and drinking swill doesn't make it right. Then, after years of horrible eating and drinking habits they join each other in a competition to see how many drugs they can stuff down their throats. Next, the complaining contests begin about all the side-effects, and more drugs are prescribed for these side-effects. Of course, they expect lots of sympathy and everyone's presence at the hospital when they have successfully destroyed themselves. This may seem harsh, but I know only too well how people—especially family members—can create great trauma and drama, because you've made a decision to follow a better way. If necessary, keep the kids always in sight when they are around. Plus, rarely, if ever, leave them alone with the spoilers. Sometimes even parents sabotage efforts made to improve dietary habits for their own child/children. Just remember, it is necessary and correct to take care of the edifices that house our souls as best as possible. That is part of the life assignment too, and kids need care.

Some kids are tough and can tolerate an occasional chance encounter with the standard American fare.

However, if you have a fair-skinned, light eyed youngster who is prone to immune distress, he/she cannot tolerate immune assaults no matter who wants to "treat" them.

So many obnoxious deeds are done, and people are programmed to accept them. For example, vaccinations are socially acceptable, since they are forced upon the public by those in control. Yet, who wants to be the parent responsible for causing vaccination-induced autism? Who also would wish to bear the grief of crib death, retardation, or cancer because of vaccinations? This may sound radical, but there is massive evidence that this happens with great frequency. Books that are required reading concerning this subject are *Saying No to Vaccines; Vaccines: The Risks, The Benefits, The Choices; Vaccines: What CDC Documents and Science Reveal;* and *FOWL!* all by Dr. Sherri Tenpenny. There is so much logical and reputable information available concerning the dangers of vaccinations, that it is surely an injustice to children to avoid reviewing it. There are many DVDs, CDs, and books that confirm the dangers of this practice. This revealing information is readily available on the internet and in books stores.

Diabetes at every age level is increasing at a shocking rate. Yet, I see parents stuffing cookies, candy, and cake down the throats of babies in strollers—getting them hooked on sugar as young as possible. Sugar is an addiction, just as surely as drugs and alcohol are. Most people hooked on the latter two were sugarholics when they were small children. They most likely had enabling family members, *who were just helping the kid have a little fun.* Even if you or those around you are addicted, for heaven's sake don't inflict that onto the children. Every generation is getting weaker, and as a result the reactions are getting more violent. In the past a few children had asthma, but rarely did they ever have severe complications. Now it is as common as colds, and kids are dying from asthma attacks. Cancer, arthritis, diabetes, AIDS, multiple sclerosis and more—all of them were once considered to be older people's diseases. Now children are more commonly afflicted than ever before. Is it God's punishment? It certainly is not. If money and industry remain more important than the human soul, this is the beginning of the end of our health and social strength. We must help each other to grow to higher levels spiritually, mentally, and physically. It must start with protecting youngsters from depravity of every sort. This includes that which is consumed to that which they are exposed to on the media and in their lives. This is the first step for a better future.

If you are reading this book, then you obviously care enough to do whatever is beneficial as much as possible. If someone gave you this book, then the children you are involved with most likely need help. Don't stop reading, because everyone needs help in some way.

Vitamin C

Scurvy led to the discovery of vitamin C. Many sailors became weak and quickly died from lack of vitamin C on long sea voyages. Vitamin C was first isolated from oranges, lemons, and potato peels—not the potato itself. It was found that the sailors responded quickly to a daily ration of one ounce of lemon or lime juice and the potato peelings as part of their rations. These foods are all still recognized as natural sources of this vitamin.

Szent Gyorgyi found that cabbage, as well as raw adrenal cortex from cows, contained considerable quantities of vitamin C. He used crude extracts of those sources in the treatment of disease with excellent results. When he made a purified extract to isolate only the vitamin C molecule, the results were negligible. This was how he determined that crude, raw vitamin C was preferred over any type of synthesized, isolated, or adulterated source. Pure, natural food source supplements are always most beneficial. Likewise, synthetic vitamins mixed in an organic food base are less beneficial than natural concentrates. This is merely an attempt to confuse consumers with cheap synthetics included in a generally recognized as desirable food base.

How vitamin C functions in the body

Vitamin C is a component of collagen, the substance that holds the body together. It is also essential for the formation and presence of healthy connective tissue. Collagen is the glue that keeps the trillions of cells that compose the body together. When it degenerates, the connective tissue—the cartilage, ligaments, and walls of the blood vessels become weak and flaccid. When this happens, viruses and bacteria can easily invade and cause disease and infections. Thus, strong connective tissue acts as a protective barrier from these invaders. Vitamin C also strengthens other natural enemy fighters in the body such as the phagocytes and antibodies. With a healthy liver and ample vitamin C, vigorous and active antibodies are produced. Active antibodies cause bacteria to become harmless. They are the defense against allergy reactions as well. Such allergies would include sensitivity to pollens, dandruff, dust, foreign proteins in food, vaccines, and serums. Some common reactions to these allergenic substances include hay fever, hives, eczema, asthma, and itching. This vitamin is most effective when given before exposure to allergens, yet it also helps relieve symptoms after contact has been made as well.

Any weakness in the tissues is a definite sign of the need for vitamin C supplementation. If the toothbrush is pink after brushing, this is a sure sign of vitamin C deficiency. Many people, including children, have what is called subclinical scurvy. This means it is not a full-blown case, but the symptoms and the destruction are chronic. Not only is the strength of the teeth and bones affected, but also the tissue surrounding the teeth will bleed when brushed. With chronic deficiency teeth and bones become soft, porous, brittle and damaged, or are easily broken. With teeth the enamel weakens, and as gums become inflamed, they recede. That is where the old saying "long in the tooth" comes from. When the supporting structure is weak, the teeth loosen. This allows bacteria and pus to build up and pyorrhea pockets form. Natural vitamin C and plenty of it is required immediately. Without action, all teeth and bone structures will be irreparably damaged. Children and teens do have symptoms of subclinical scurvy, and they may even lose permanent teeth at a young age.

Stress is another major factor that increases the need for vitamin C. If a child is accident prone, two issues are evident. First of all this is an indication of weakened adrenal glands. The adrenal glands are the "coping mechanism" of the body, and they require the highest quantity of vitamin C in the entire body. A low-carbohydrate diet with plenty of protein, essential fatty acids, and whole, fresh, raw, low-sugar fruit and vegetables will improve the status of the adrenals. As well, the intake of a teaspoonful or more of a kid's formula royal jelly/pumpkinseed oil along with natural vitamin C are important supplements every day.

Secondly, while the frequency of accidents and injuries will lessen once the adrenals are functioning better, the accident prone child needs vitamin C and adequate protein to heal injuries faster.

Strong collagen is particularly important in the prevention and eradication of disease. Good collagen integrity is especially effective for tuberculosis and stomach ulcers. It helps to prevent further breakdown of the tissues and retards reinfection. Yes, tuberculosis is once again on the rise. Adequate precautions and good health practices should be observed to protect the family from exposure. Anyone who flies and is in busy public areas has an opportunity to contract tuberculosis and other serious diseases. Then, these diseases can be passed on to others. There is a far greater chance of being infected with a serious disease than a terrorist attack from a third world country. Think how easily children share illnesses when they attend day care and school. Therefore, these dreadfully contagious diseases are easily spread among children as well as adults.

The many needs for vitamin C

Capillaries are hair-sized blood vessels that permeate every part of the body. These capillaries bring nourishment and oxygen to the cells to keep the body alive and beautifully functioning. They also remove waste products. Without enough vitamin C the capillaries become fragile and break down. When this occurs, blood leaks into the tissues, bone marrow, joints, gums, and so on. This leads to rheumatic disease and other ailments.

When the body's capillary system is depleted and the cells' food supply is eliminated, the cells quickly die. These dead cells become a breeding ground for bacteria, which can then damage the joints, kidneys, and heart.

Two common signs of fragile capillaries are nose bleeds and easy bruising. Food rich in vitamin C must be added to the diet as well as supplements from a natural form of vitamin C to help stop these symptoms.

Vitamin C is required for many functions in the body. The following are examples of the many ways the body uses this important vitamin:

Requirement	Function of vitamin C
thyroid gland	production of metabolic hormones and health of the gland
adrenal glands	for efficiency of the glands and production of hormones
pituitary	health of the master gland/for the production of hormones
iron	retention and utilization of iron in the body and for prevention of anemia
folic acid	needed to convert folic acid to its usable form (for treating megaloblastic anemia)
amino acids	for the activation of tyrosine, proline, and phenylalanine; for tissue and collagen formation
blood vessels	strengthens all vessels/prevents painful bruising, bad veins, and blood spots on the skin

eyes	high concentration in vitreous fluid, lens, iris, retina, and cornea; prevents damage and eye diseases
cardiovascular	acts as a diuretic; aids in the excretion of excess water through urine; improves capillary health

The function of the entire endocrine system is dependent upon vitamin C. The endocrine glands and the brain, liver, kidneys, pancreas, thymus, and spleen require the greatest concentrations of this vitamin in the body. Without enough vitamin C there are many negative effects on the developing child. The results are a lack or shortage of important hormones and, thus, a failure to thrive and grow in an appropriate manner. There is more vitamin C in children's actively multiplying cells and tissues than there is in adult tissues. Needless to say, it is an important component to include in their diets every day, since it is easily lost in perspiration and urine. It is easy to tell when the adrenals are weak, because as mentioned previously they are the "coping glands." When a child's behavior is difficult to tolerate and he/she is highly emotional—screaming, crying, tantrums, angry outbursts, whining and moodiness—the child most certainly needs adrenal support. Remember, children need daily sources of natural vitamin C, because they are growing and developing. Particularly during growth spurts, they need even more.

Other vitamin C deficiencies are also very common among children today. These include inability to sleep, poor concentration, allergies, asthma, poor eyesight (along with lack of chromium), anemia, bleeding gums and poor dentition, easy bruising, susceptibility to infections, fevers, blood sugar swings, childhood arthritis and joint/bone abnormalities, slow wound healing, and poor collagen formation (note: collagen is the glue that holds the cells together). If a child is sensitive to cold or hot temperatures and loud noises startle or frighten him/her, a natural, raw vitamin C supplement will help resolve the problem. Sweetened artificial forms of vitamin C are not recommended. Any ascorbic acid supplement is a synthetic form of vitamin C.

Vitamin C losses and requirements

Vitamin C is easily destroyed by oxygen, alkaline substances, and high temperatures. Other losses occur from inhalation of toxic substances such as smoke, pesticides, fumes from gasoline, lead paints, cleaning solvents, and smog. Drugs, such as aspirin, barbiturates, insulin, thyroid extract, antihistamines, adrenaline, and asthma drugs, deplete vitamin C. If hydrochloric acid is lacking in the stomach, vitamin C absorption is inhibited.

When allergic shock or chemical poisoning occur, vitamin C is hugely effective in both prevention of the reaction and in the cure. It supports liver function in detoxification of perilous chemicals such as lead, bromide, gasoline, arsenic, and many other chemicals commonly used today.

In today's toxic world the most minimal amount of vitamin C for babies is 50 mg, while children and teens require at least 100 to 150 mg per day. Much more is needed during highly stressful times for women during pregnancy and for the reversal of toxic exposure or allergy reaction.

Vitamin C on the retail store shelves, including health food stores, is mainly produced from synthetic sources. Synthetic forms should not be used. Ascorbic acid is usually synthesized from corn and, thus, is contaminated with GMOs. For health and safety do not buy anything made from genetically modified material.

Food straight from the garden is always the best source of nutrients, and I cannot recommend enough that everyone should have a garden or even container gardens if there is no room for planting. All plants should be grown from heirloom organic seeds that are found in health food stores or at some better nurseries. It will save lots of money on groceries, and the entire family will be better nourished. Kids can help. They can choose which food plants they would like to sow and, ultimately, eat. Then they can help water the garden, watch the plants grow, and practice weeding and pruning. This may require supervision for young children and inexperienced adults. There are organic gardening and container gardening books that will make this learning project fun and easy.

While waiting for that garden to grow, buy only organic food which is produced locally whenever possible. Get it as fresh as you can, because exposure to air and light, extended storage time, and cooking/heat destroy much of the nutrient content of foods. For example, a good source of vitamin C is fresh organic oranges. However, fresh-squeezed orange juice should be drunk immediately. The longer it stands the more vitamin C is lost. Commercial pasteurized juice has little to no natural vitamin C. Vegetables and fruits stored at room temperature lose much of their vitamin C after just a few days. That's right, straight off the tree or vine at the peak of ripeness is the ideal. Eating food raw or vegetables steamed just until tender is always best. Some foods, like broccoli and cauliflower, need to be steamed just until the color starts to change and brighten. Otherwise, they have spicules, which are indigestible.

Fresh, organic, mostly raw food is the key to good health for the whole family. There is little nourishment from the standard boxed and canned food. Because of this, many people, including children, feel depleted. They are tired, weak, mentally impaired, full of aches and pain, and suffer from health issues galore. When the entire family is well nourished, there are far less crises, sickness, and bad behavior. The entire family is happier, calmer and more physically, mentally, and spiritually balanced.

Natural food sources of vitamin C

Excellent sources of vitamin C include red bell pepper, parsley, broccoli, papaya, strawberries, oranges, lemons, grapefruit, cantaloupe, kiwi fruit, cauliflower, kale, mustard greens, collard greens, romaine lettuce, Brussels sprouts, turnip greens, cabbage, tomatoes, chard, raspberries, asparagus, celery, spinach, fennel, pineapple, watermelon, green beans, cranberries, and all types of summer squash. Very good sources include cucumber, ground cloves, all varieties of winter squash, blueberries, carrots, garlic, apricots, calf's liver, sweet potatoes, plums, green peas, onions, chili peppers, and potatoes. Good sources are basil, cayenne pepper, oregano, leeks, yams, bananas, apples, beets, shiitake mushrooms, Bartlett pears, Concord grapes, yellow corn, and avocado. Organic or wild are always best.

One of my favorite vitamin C recipes is so fast and easy to make that it is almost shocking that it is so nutritious and tasty. Even for those who do not like to cook or really understand how to cook, this is so easy a child could make this. Why not let them?

Avo-Cream Dip, Mayonnaise, or Salad Dressing

1 medium avocado, peeled and cut into pieces
6 to 8 cherry tomatoes, washed
1 small onion or 2 green onions, washed and cut into pieces
2 tablespoons black seed spice oil
2 tablespoons Austrian pumpkinseed oil/rosemary oil mixture
4 tablespoons crude cold-pressed Turkish sesame seed oil
4 tablespoons rice vinegar
1 tablespoon capers
1 tablespoon oregano herb and spice mixture
1 teaspoon sea salt

Put the above ingredients into a blender, and blend until smooth and creamy. Avo-Cream may be used as a dip for vegetables or chips, a spread on crackers, mayonnaise substitute on bread for sandwiches, or make a lovely vitamin C-rich green salad, and use it as a dressing. It may be a sauce over meat or cooked vegetables. Consume soon after making so that the nutrients are fully utilized and enjoyed.

Fresh fruity fruit

Another quick and painless recipe is to cut fresh fruit (choose from those on the vitamin C list) into chunks and squeeze fresh orange juice over the fruit. The vitamin C in the orange juice keeps the fruit from oxidizing, so it looks and stays fresh and appetizing. Again, prepare and eat as soon as possible. This makes a great dessert or breakfast dish that most everyone will love. For the little ones or the whole family just blend a small avocado, 1/3 cup of papaya, and 1/3 cup of mango until smooth. It makes a creamy and yummy pudding type of dessert. This may be poured over fresh fruit as a topping. I use the Bullet Blender every day for simple recipes that are delicious, fast, and nourishing. Create your own, and let the children help.

Bioflavonoids

Like vitamin C, bioflavonoids are important for the circulatory system. They act as antioxidants, and they protect the capillaries in the body far more effectively than vitamin C. The capillaries carry the nutrients to even the most obscure cells. When the capillaries weaken and the veins become porous, disease develops rapidly. The red corpuscles can actually pass through the porous blood vessels, and the individual may suffer from problems such as easy bruising, nose bleeds, blood in the urine, rectal bleeding, and hemorrhoids.

The capillaries are extremely fine, and they are plentiful. If all the capillaries were removed from a single average-sized man and placed end to end, they would wrap around the world two and a half times. Since children are much smaller, this would be reduced. However, even they have thousands of miles of capillaries, which need daily nourishment. The capillaries, veins, and arteries need nourishment to be strong and supple, because they are the transport system to every cell and organ in the body for all substances in the blood such as hormones and nutrients from food including oxygen and water. They also remove waste material from the breakdown products of metabolism and any toxic substances from disease, injury, or environmental exposure. Healthy capillaries mean that the body will fight infections rapidly and thoroughly. That is why all diseases respond favorably when the millions of miles of capillaries are strengthened with the addition of bioflavonoids in the daily diet.

Other known actions of bioflavonoids are their powerful anti-inflammatory and antibiotic benefits. Thus, they are useful for the prevention and/or treatment of colds, cold sores, rheumatic fever, allergies, arthritis, diabetes, bacterial infections, many eye problems, hemorrhages, toxicity from drugs, and much more. They also act as a detoxifier from drug damage, benzene, chlorinated hydrocarbons, arsenic, and other poisons.

Bioflavonoids function in concert with vitamin C. Concentrated forms of natural bioflavonoids in combination with natural vitamin C are available. Look for children's formulas which are purely natural plant sources.

Bioflavonoid sources and requirements

There are bioflavonoids in many foods. These foods also contain vitamin C. Lemons, oranges, and paprika from red peppers are good examples of this, especially the organic ones. The organic sources are richer in nutrients and, therefore, a better buy. All bioflavonoids help prevent capillary bleeding. Other food sources are grapes, black currants, gooseberries, and rose hips. This type of fruit bioflavonoid is called hesperidin. Buckwheat supplies another biologically active bioflavonoid called rutin. Rutin is also found in eucalyptus and wild berries. There are many other bioflavonoids, but quercitrin and quercetin are commonly known.

In citrus fruit the pulp and the white substance directly under the peel are the sources of bioflavonoids. Fresh squeezed juice from organic sun-ripened citrus fruit will provide delicious vitamin C, and the pulp and slices of the citrus fruit left to soak in the juice will enrich it with bioflavonoids.

Children would greatly benefit from ingesting 50 to 100 mgs of bioflavonoids daily with the same ratio of natural C. Bioflavonoids prevent the oxidation of vitamin C. Since they work together, it is wise to use the natural combination of the two.

FAT SOLUBLE VITAMINS

The fat soluble vitamins are A, D, E, and K. To utilize these vitamins in the body some consumption of fat is necessary. Low-fat diets compromise the intake and storage of these important nutrients. Also avoid the use of mineral oil internally and externally, because it blocks the absorption of fat soluble vitamins.

Fat soluble vitamins are stored in the body longer than the water soluble vitamins. Therefore, signs of depletion of these nutrients may take longer to occur. As always natural vitamins from food sources are preferable to synthetic, and megadoses are not necessary unless there are established deficiency symptoms.

Vitamin A

Vitamin A was one of the first vitamins discovered. In 1904 cod liver oil was used for treating conjunctivitis in Japan. Other studies showed promise when rats with conjunctivitis were successfully healed with milk and butter. Yet, it wasn't until 1913 when it was finally determined that a substance from fat contained the healing properties. In 1917 McCollum and Simmonds named this substance vitamin A.

Vitamin A is highly important for immune function. The health of the skin and epithelium are dependent upon this important nutrient. The epithelial lining includes the cells that line the nose, sinuses, mouth, throat, bronchial tubes, lungs, stomach, intestines, gallbladder, urinary tract and bladder, kidneys, mastoids, inner ear, inner surface of the eyelids, and conjunctiva. Healthy skin and epithelium act as barriers for bacteria and other infectious agents. Sufficient vitamin A prevents infection of those susceptible areas mentioned and helps to protect the body from disease, even cancer.

Healthy epithelial cells multiply at a normal pace, because they secrete moisture. Cells deficient in vitamin A are also deficient in moisture. They multiply too fast, then die, becoming hard and dry. The cells below them continue the same process and push up the hard, dry dead cells above them. This forms layers of dead cells called dandruff. Even household pets have this problem when their diets are deficient in vitamin A.

Bacteria love to hide and feed on the dead, dry matter, and they excrete an enzyme which is toxic to the body. This enzyme breaks down the body's cells and causes inflammation.

Healthy cells replete with vitamin A fight bacteria with anti-enzymes. Lysozyme is such an anti-enzyme found in the mucus in the nose and tears. It acts as a strong antiseptic, and vitamin A is needed for the production of this substance.

Animals seem to respond faster to vitamin A treatment than humans. There is usually a noticeable improvement in about five days. Response time for humans is generally longer, with the length of time depending on the degree of deficiency. Vitamin A is so important that any not immediately utilized is stored in the liver for future use.

Eyes and vitamin A

Besides conjunctivitis (commonly known as pink eye in children) night blindness is also a sign of vitamin A deficiency. There is a substance in the retina of the eye called visual purple. The eye uses some of the visual purple when light enters it, and this tells the brain what the eye is seeing. This visual purple is constantly replaced by the body as it is used if vitamin A and protein are available. If not, night blindness/poor vision in dim light occurs.

Sties are increasingly common among children and adults. They are a sure sign of vitamin A deficiency as are corneal ulcers, severely itchy, burning eyes, and even excessive eye blinking and squinting. For eye infections vitamins A and B_2 are particularly beneficial. Any child who has sties and other eye infections must have vitamin A included in the diet, and supplemental sources should be considered.

Vitamin A protects the eyes from damage and potential blindness. During childhood illnesses stores of this vitamin are rapidly diminished. Therefore, with such diseases as measles the eyes may be damaged and even blindness may result, especially if the child is already deficient in vitamin A. If during illness the child complains about the light hurting his/her eyes, there is, no doubt, a deficiency in vitamin A. Also, a B_2 deficiency is likely. Vitamin A is mandatory for good eyesight in children and for the elimination of eye defects in infants. Organic butter, cream, and egg yolk are the easiest and tastiest ways to increase vitamin A in the diet on a daily basis for children as well as expectant and lactating mothers. The Polar-source wild sockeye salmon oil is an excellent source of natural vitamin A. Available in an 8-ounce liquid and 500 mg fish gelatin capsules this is the ideal, complete fish oil supplement for children. All the important unrefined factors of fish oil are present, plus natural vitamin A, vitamin D, and astaxanthin, which is a powerful carotenoid, are available. This certainly makes it more beneficial and cost effective than even food sources.

Hair, skin, and nails

As mentioned earlier signs and symptoms are very important indicators of health status. Years ago some family doctors recognized various signs of vitamin A deficiency. They examined patients carefully and asked many questions. Now invasive tests are more common, because nutrition isn't taken seriously. Furthermore, it is a litigious society, and patient processing is fast paced. Unfortunately, drugs are automatically prescribed as the treatment of choice in most situations, even for nutritional deficiency symptoms. The following are some of the common signs and symptoms of vitamin A deficiency. To be able to recognize these health abnormalities early is beneficial for the entire family.

hair	dry and coarse (same as hypothyroid); no shine or natural luster; unusual amount of falling hair
scalp	itchy for no apparent reason; dandruff

nails	brittle, peeling, or break easily; heavy vertical line down the center of the nail
skin	clogged pores-blackheads, whiteheads, pimples, and other skin blemishes (acne); oil glands do not function properly; bumps like gooseflesh on the back of the arms, elbows, knees, buttocks, and thighs; dry skin susceptible to boils, carbuncles, impetigo, cysts and eczema

The most common storage site for vitamin A is in the liver. However, a small amount is found in the kidneys and lungs. Of course, children naturally cannot store as much as an adult, and babies have little to no storage capacity. Years ago Dr. Wolback at the Harvard School of Medicine stated that babies should be given fish liver oil immediately after they are born instead of waiting until they are six to eight weeks old. This is not commonly done today, but it is even more important now than ever. Regrettably, ocean contaminants are so prolific that most fish liver oils are heavily refined. When this occurs, much of the natural vitamin A and D are lost. Some manufacturers add synthetic vitamins and other ingredients to fortify their refined fish liver oil supplements. Again, naturally occurring nutrients are always superior and safer choices than synthetic ones.

For a period of time even eggs were eliminated from the American diet. Actually, this isn't such a bad idea, if the chickens are fed the "mad pellets." These pellets contain the guts and pieces of dead animals and dead chickens from commercial processing plants. Eggs from organic free-range chickens are the kind to use. Even if they are a little more expensive, they are more nutritious and safer to eat. (Remember you cast a vote for the type of food you are willing to tolerate with every penny you spend.) Also, vitamin A is only in the yolk of the egg. It was fashionable for awhile to throw away the yolk, when the cholesterol scare was being touted. However, it is reasonable to use the complete organic egg in some way every day, especially when there is a possibility of a vitamin A deficiency. For the most absorption of important nutrients, don't overcook the egg. The yolk should be somewhat runny. Eggs within recipes are included as part of daily egg consumption. A variety of eggs may be used. Quail and duck eggs are relatively common and may cause fewer allergic reactions.

Preventive uses of vitamin A

Vitamin A stores are rapidly exhausted when diseases occur affecting the liver, kidneys, intestines, and respiratory system. The body's requirement increases as the availability decreases. Thus, if it is not replenished, inflammation and illnesses, such as cirrhosis, renal failure, pneumonia, bronchitis, and other ailments, will progress rapidly.

As vitamin A deficiency continues to increase, kidney and bladder stones are becoming more common even among children. This increases the incidence of infection, because the stones impede waste removal/urine flow. Rats deprived of butter and milk soon developed stones in the bladder. If you are using synthetic food, like margarine, fake/refined packaged meals such as some of the macaroni and cheese dinners, and little fresh food, no doubt there will be negative consequences.

Children need vitamin A for proper growth. In other words the bone structure of the body is forming, as are the teeth and enamel. If there is a failure to thrive and develop appropriately, there is a definite nutrition connection.

Especially during the first years of life and also continuing through the teen years the health and structure of the individual is established both physically and mentally for the rest of his/her life. Vitamins play a major role in that development, and deficiency in vitamin A shows up in many ways. For example, allergic reactions are common in the vitamin A-deficient child. Usually, dark circles under the eyes are a sign that the child is eating something which is causing a reaction. Again, remember to check the back of the arms for those telltale bumps. Warts may also be a common aggravation. Chronic ear infections and colds are also vitamin A deficiency signals, as is chronic body odor which is evident even after a bath. For many health problems associated with vitamin A deficiency, zinc may be a requirement as well. White spots on the fingernails are always an indicator of a need for both zinc and vitamin A.

Does your child drive you wild at the dinner table with whining and crying and refusing to eat? (How often does your family eat at the dinner table?) Just as thiamine depletion adversely affects a child's appetite, so does insufficient vitamin A. Always think of this when there is a "fussy eater" in the house. Then, the next step is to create as many ways as possible to get nutrient-dense foods into his/her tummy. It is easier on both child and parents, if this is a game instead of a fight. One woman I know was almost an adult before she found out that the "trees" she had been eating for so many years were also called broccoli. Fussy eaters use tactics to control the eating part of their lives. If parents make a huge issue of it, they become even more stubborn and rebellious. Yet, when they push for the goodies, they should be reminded that healthy food comes first. When good food is consumed, they are then allowed a healthy treat.

Parents must abide by the rules too, or they won't take those guidelines concerning eating habits seriously. Most people somewhat follow their parents' examples, unless there have been major changes in lifestyles. There are so many benefits for the whole family, when such a discipline is followed to include better health, more stability, and happiness. Well-nourished children have far fewer problems and emotional issues than those who eat what is the commonly accepted fare. Many parents are reporting that the children who have only junk food are clamoring to trade lunches with their children for the more healthy food. Studies show it is a normal instinct for a child to seek food that is nourishing. Unfortunately, over time with the constant barrage of the media and peer group pressure this natural instinct is eventually extinguished.

Vitamin A sources and requirements

Vitamin A is extremely important for children's immune systems, growth, beauty, and well-being. The best and most natural sources are from burbot or sockeye salmon oil, liver, cream, butter, egg yolk, and milk. They are the easiest sources to obtain and include in meals and snacks. Make an effort to use organic sources whenever possible.

There are no vegetable sources of vitamin A. The only young children I have seen with severely dry and coarse hair were vegans—meaning no meat, eggs, or dairy. After following a vegan diet for several years, a lady had to relent and take Polar-source sockeye salmon oil, when she began to lose her eye sight. This was due to insufficient vitamin A. Even though she ate all types of vegetables, beta carotene does not support the body in the same way as vitamin A. Also, some people are not able to convert beta carotene into vitamin A, especially those with blood sugar problems and thyroid conditions. It is especially important for children to get all the nourishment that they need while growing and developing, and the vegan diet does not provide enough protein, B_{12}, vitamin A, vitamin D, and perhaps other factors as well. At least when dairy, eggs, fish liver oil, and royal jelly are included in children's diets, they usually have fewer problems.

The fast food, junk food routine for the busy family is even far worse. These kids are getting little or nothing of any value, and actually are harmed by the hydrogenated oils, sugar/synthetic sweeteners, food dyes, and other chemicals that are in such refined worthless products or that which is so-called food. Synthetic food will not nourish your child, nor will synthetic vitamins and improper/inadequate mineral sources. Buy organic prepared fresh vegetables and meats if you are in such a hurry or don't know how to cook. Parents need healthy fuel too. Humans are creatures of habit, and people are brainwashed by advertisements to use the "in" or "hot" items and to desire food and drinks which may or may not be good for them. These companies know that children become accustomed to certain smells, textures, and tastes that will be the foundation of their future food choices and desires. This is how they develop customers for life, and how the natural inborn ability that every child has to make good food selections is overwhelmed.

Now, how much vitamin A is necessary for superbly good health? Well, those who are supposedly in the know keep revising and dropping the minimum daily requirements. Always keep in mind the word minimum. It means just enough to survive. Yet, is merely surviving good enough for any family? It was advised until fairly recently that from day one babies should consume 6000 IU of natural (not synthetic) vitamin A daily. There is an established history of successfully using this practice, and the babies thrived. Mothers who nurse should take no less than 10,000 IU daily. The growing child certainly requires 10,000 IU, and the optimal amount could be as high as 20,000 IU or more depending on symptoms or ill health. When a child is frequently sick, the requirement is greater. Do keep in mind the fat soluble vitamins are stored in the body, and an overdose could occur if large amounts of vitamin A (50,000 IU plus) are taken over a prolonged period. Symptoms of overdose are similar to deficiency symptoms. Headache beginning in the back of the neck and extending up to the eyes is a major symptom.

The only concern with fish liver oil as a vitamin supplement is that most of it is highly processed due to the toxicity of the water where the fish live. Somehow, the poor creatures manage to survive but not without consequences. Formerly, the processing was minor, so many of the co-factors that work with vitamin A were also present. Then, overdosing was exceedingly rare. The more refined anything is the less true value it represents for the nourishment of the body. The probability of toxicity also increases. Since vitamin A is commonly eliminated in highly refined fish liver oils, synthetic sources may be added until the vitamin A level reaches a credible amount for the label. This may not be revealed, since the claim is synthetic and natural are the same. This is dangerous, because the body will not tolerate synthetic A the same as it does the natural form. One brand of fish oil from Alaskan sockeye salmon and a new fermented burbot (fresh water cod) oil are not refined. Due to the pristine habitat, these fish oils have no toxins. They contain substantial doses of natural vitamin A and D, all of the other natural beneficial substances such as EPA, DHA, all of the omega-3s, plus astaxanthin in the sockeye salmon oil and vitamin K in the burbot oil.

Beta carotene

Natural beta carotene is an important antioxidant. While it is often regarded as a replacement for vitamin A, it may also have different functions. Its immune-enhancing activity and its promotion of appropriate cell-to-cell communication are two notable findings. This is an important advance for the prevention and treatment of diseases such as heart disease and cancer.

Beta carotene does seem to be mandatory for skin problems. It has been shown to improve difficult cases of acne, psoriasis and eczema, and dry skin. No doubt, it does have similar actions as vitamin A.

A diet sufficient in the good, natural sources of beta carotene must also provide vitamin A-rich animal fats and cold-pressed vegetable oils to increase the flow of bile for beta carotene to be utilized by the body. The vegetable oils, especially those high in polyunsaturates, must contain antioxidants to prevent the destruction of the carotenes. Antioxidant spice oils, such as rosemary, oregano, sage, and coriander, are preferable to the synthetic chemical antioxidants such as BHA and BHT. The bile salts stimulated by fats and oils and certain fat-splitting enzymes work together in the small intestine to produce what is called pro-vitamin A from beta carotene. It must be noted that individuals with health issues, such as digestive impairment, thyroid disease, liver disease, or diabetes, cannot convert beta carotene to vitamin A. Even if the body is able to achieve conversion of pro-vitamin A, a huge amount of fruit and vegetables must be consumed to meet the most minimal vitamin A requirement. Getting children to eat any vegetables may take a supreme effort, let alone large quantities on a daily basis.

Pro-vitamin A is not actually retinol, which is the animal source of vitamin A. It is unfortunate that there is such a dearth of research in nutrition, since we do not have a complete understanding of how these nutrients function, how they are alike, and how they differ. The medical industry has no interest in this vast scientific wonder of foods, nutrients, and their relationship to the human body.

Synthetic sources of beta carotene in supplements have not had a good review. They may actually cause more harm than good, so some research studies indicate.

Sources of beta carotene

Major sources of this powerful antioxidant are from beet and turnip greens, carrots, sweet potatoes, romaine lettuce, collard greens, dandelion greens, kale, kohlrabi, parsley, cilantro, spinach, winter squash, broccoli, apricots, and cantaloupe. Since the sources of beta carotene are mainly from fruit, vegetables, and algae, the only major reaction seems to be that the skin turns yellow to orange when there is a beta carotene overload. This is unlikely to happen with children, unless they are taking a large supplement dose. If it did happen, just reduce or eliminate the source. Natural foods are not likely to ever be a problem.

A great way to get children to consume enough beta carotene is to make fresh juice every day. Use the foods previously mentioned, and try different combinations. Enjoy the juice immediately after making it to retain the highest amount of nutrients. Teach the kids how to feed the carrots and greens into the juicer, and how to safely use the plunger to help the process. Children are more likely to experiment with new foods if they play a part in the preparation. Fresh pineapple, papaya, mango, and frozen banana are nice to mix with the greens, because it would be the rare child who would enjoy the green juice alone. The first three fruits have enzymes which help with digestion. There is nothing complex about making juice. Select the freshest organic vegetables and fruit you can find, wash them well, some you may need to peel, then juice them and drink immediately to get the greatest amount of nourishment.

I always use about a teaspoon of the seeds from the papaya, since they are full of enzymes. However, I do not recommend using apple, pear, and citrus seeds. They contain potentially toxic substances.

Vitamin D

In 1919 vitamin D was discovered to be the sunshine vitamin. It was found in cod liver oil, which was used to cure rickets. Rickets is a bone malformation disease in children. While many people think that this disease no longer occurs, toddlers frequently have bowed legs. This is a sure sign of rickets and a need for vitamin D. Improvements have been noted with the consumption of fresh summer butter and eggs. Plus, unrefined Polar fish liver/Alaskan sockeye salmon oil, burbot liver oil, and sunshine are also reliable solutions.

In cities with heavy cloud cover, fog, smog, haze and lots of rain a higher incidence of rickets is recorded. However, I've seen toddlers with rickets (severely bowed legs) in sunny south Texas as well as northern Manitoba. One place was too hot to go out in the sun and the other too cold. Fish liver oil, such as Alaskan sockeye salmon and burbot oil, or animal liver are the best options for such situations. Black- and brown-skinned children need more sun exposure, since the additional melanin in the skin reduces natural vitamin D synthesis. A low-cholesterol diet is also detrimental. Cholesterol is the key substance in the production of vitamin D in the body.

Vitamin D and dental development

After extensive research May Mellanby discovered that even a mild form of rickets had a major impact on the development of teeth in infants. It also affected the conformation of the jawbone. Thus, the children ultimately had narrow dental arches and crooked, over-lapping, and protruding teeth. Other complications, such as defective bite and faulty alignment of the teeth, affected chewing and digestion. Additionally, dental caries were prolific. Gum infections were also a factor.

Dr. Weston Price was a dentist who traveled all over the world studying the health and dentition of children. Those in remote villages living under primitive conditions with limited food choices fared much better than those in the cities with a wide selection of prepared foods. It can only be that fresh air, sunshine, no chemicals, and no so-called civilized lifestyles are physically beneficial components. The children he encountered had beautiful, well-formed teeth, dental arches with no crowding or malformation of the teeth, strong jawbones, and no dental caries. For further information, newsletter, book list, and membership inquiries view the website www.ppnf.org or call the non-profit Price-Pottenger Nutrition Foundation in California at 1-800-366-3748.

For healthy dentition even newborns need exposure to sunlight. For a daily supply of vitamins A and D cod liver oil and/or halibut liver oil are common supplemental sources. Yet, the finest sources are derived from certain natural wild sockeye salmon and burbot. Most fish oils are highly refined due to toxicity of polluted waters and high mercury levels in the fish. Burbot oil and a specific sockeye salmon oil are derived from the cleanest sources left on the planet. They have not been exposed to the harsh detergents and elaborate cleaning processes and chemicals, which remove many of the important factors of the natural oil. Most spectacularly, they contain all the important essential fatty acids and vitamins A and D, plus other natural components that are virtually unknown. Also, they are unique, because they are ethically harvested, and there is no waste.

Nursing mothers most likely need to supplement with vitamin D daily, unless they are in the sun every day or use fresh water fish liver oils. Fresh water fish may soon be one of the few reliable sources of vitamins A and D. The oceans are at risk for two reasons. One reason is that they have become the world toilet and trash depository. Many years ago it was decided that "the solution to pollution is dilution," and that the amount of water in the oceans is so vast that it just couldn't matter. Unfortunately, contamination is so rampant, that now it matters. The second terrifying fact was revealed in the *London Times*. On October 2006 British researchers stated that by 2048 certain species of the edible types of fish most commonly used today would be extinct. Alarmingly, it is occurring much faster than the projected date. This is due to dire pollution, crude oil contamination, and the fishing factory ships that vacuum all life forms out of the water. Whatever is caught is caught. If it is the type of fish they want to sell, it is sold. The rest of the unfortunate creatures are destroyed. Little to no breeding stock is left to replenish the oceans. The quality and quantity of fish are already so depleted that, as mentioned previously, the highly refined fish liver oil is being stealthily fortified with synthetic A and D. Therefore, our favorite old standbys are not dependable sources any longer. With so much toxic gunk in the fish, the refining processes that remove these poisons destroy much of the naturally occurring health-giving substances that our bodies need. Further, some claim that around 100 gallons of health food-grade fish oil is required to make a mere one gallon of ultrarefined or pharmaceutical-grade fish oil. With these practices, we can bid the fish population (and fish supplements) goodbye unless these destructive actions are stopped now. That is why the wild, remote-source Polar sockeye salmon oil and the fresh water cod liver (burbot) oil are so important, because these naturally pure oils are from well-managed stocks, which are not depleted.

How vitamin D works

Vitamin D is more of a hormone than a vitamin. It regulates the enzyme phosphatase, which essentially controls the formation of bone. This enzyme detaches the phosphorus molecule from fats and sugars. Once this is accomplished it unites with calcium from the blood. Then, this combination of minerals (also tiny amounts of other minerals as well) go to work to build bone and the skeletal structure. Then, this structure is hardened. Little children have very flexible bones which are substantially collagen. If vitamin D is deficient, deformity occurs. Then, when the bones solidify, any structural damage will be permanent. Thus, pain and injury are forever part of the individual's life.

If the minerals that make up bone are deficient, especially calcium and phosphorus, growth will be stunted and bone malformations will occur. Today, a junk food diet low in minerals and too little vitamin D spells disaster for many children, and the numbers are growing. There are more children now who are developing curvature of the spine. Then, chronic infection such as tuberculosis may settle into this weakened area. Also, recent evidence indicates that parasites in the spinal fluid may play a role in the spinal deformity. Unfortunately, modern medicine's treatment of choice is to surgically insert a metal rod or rods in the spine and, thus, try to straighten it in this most barbaric and painful manner. Supplementing with vitamin D and the appropriate minerals and using a treatment called the rain drop therapy has provided significant results. All of this is non-invasive and painless. Rain drop therapy consists of rubbing the spine with certain essential plant oils, and it is proving to be very beneficial. It is not particularly a quick fix, and it takes effort to rub the oils on the spine for an extended period of time. Yet, it certainly is worth trying before submitting to such draconian action as the rod implants.

There are other symptoms of vitamin D deficiency besides the spinal deformity. This includes bowed legs, knock knees, receding chin and abnormal dental arches and teeth. Babies and toddlers with bulging foreheads are certainly deficient as well. Natural vitamin D used soon enough can correct these abnormalities. However, to absorb vitamin D into the blood, fat must be present. Thus, low fat, no fat diets are unacceptable if fat soluble vitamins are to be absorbed and utilized in the body.

Another activity of vitamin D is to charge the body with energy. Keep in mind that vitamin D causes the phosphatase enzyme to release the mineral phosphorus from fat and sugar. Then, this released phosphorus plays a major role in the blood sugar mechanism. Thus, blood sugar reaches the liver and is stored there as glycogen. Blood sugar and glycogen are converted to energy as needed, but this cannot happen when vitamin D is deficient and phosphorus is missing. Then, fatigue may be constant, because the blood sugar cannot combine with the phosphorus, which would normally carry it through the intestinal wall or to the liver. That is why a daily dose of sunshine or good fish liver oil, such as the burbot oil or the unfiltered Alaskan sockeye salmon oil, is so important.

Researchers conducted an experiment to demonstrate how critical vitamin D is for creating physical energy. They gave vitamin D to hibernating animals, after their normal blood levels had decreased as winter approached. When the hedgehogs' blood levels of vitamin D were elevated, they again became quite active and could not hibernate. Interestingly, children who play in the sun for many hours each day frequently do not require as many hours of sleep as they otherwise would.

Children who sleep excessively are likely to be deficient in vitamin D. Seasonal Affective Disorder (SAD) is the response to diminishing hours of sunlight and less vitamin D. As fall progresses into winter some children have trouble waking, are low in energy, and gain weight. Vitamin D plus the special light boxes can help alleviate these problematic symptoms. Using this light box for twenty minutes at the same time every day helps decrease symptoms of SAD. I used such a light box for a number of years while conducting business in my home office. When I turned it on, my kitty, Bartholomew, would curl up beside it and fall asleep. Then, after a time he would sit up, yawn, and leave. It seemed to be about the same time every day, so I began timing him. Sure enough he would stay in front of the box for almost exactly twenty minutes. Frequently, I would forget and sit in front of it for more than an hour. Then, the result is sort of like drinking several cups of coffee. So, I learned that when Bartholomew decided to leave, it was time to turn off the light box. If you don't have a cat that knows how to use a full-spectrum light box properly, it is probably a good idea to get a unit that has a built-in timer.

For children who lack energy it is likely necessary to supply some form of vitamin D (supplements and/or dietary sources). Remember that vitamin D is needed to get phosphorus and sugar into the muscles rather than spilling blood sugar in the urine. Also, this vitamin causes the blood to maintain a normal range of sugar, rather than being elevated. Without vitamin D the liver cannot store the excess sugar as glycogen, and the physical energy of the individuals suffers from this incomplete absorption of glycogen.

Childhood diabetes is on the increase—not only juvenile diabetes but also Type II. Type II was once common only among adults. A high sugar, nutritionally deficient diet is no doubt the major contributor to this dilemma. Sugar cravings increase when vitamin D is deficient and also when fungal overgrowth is present within the body. When the diet is changed to a healthy one and beneficial food supplements are added, the fungus is destroyed. When an appropriate amount of nutrients are maintained, even juvenile diabetes is easier to manage and, perhaps, eliminate in some cases.

The eyes are always affected by blood sugar imbalances. Vitamin D and natural chromium are both important for good eye health and vision. Research studies showed that animals suffered the same vision impairment that is common among children and adults when they have a deficiency in these nutrients. The eyes have an inability to bend light rays sufficiently, and this is called nearsightedness or myopia.

The sun offers everyone a free gift of vitamin D. During the summer only about five minutes of light a day will provide the needed amount, when the sun is thirty degrees or more above the horizon. However, during the winter in severely polluted areas or areas with plentiful rain and cloud cover, more than three hours of natural light are needed daily to keep children free from rickets. Unfortunately, in some cases there are little to no ultraviolet rays even in the out-of-doors.

Even when ultraviolet rays are available, they are easily blocked. For some unknown reason most people wear dark clothes in the winter. Heavy dark clothes and even window glass block important vitamin D-promoting rays. Lighter skinned people more readily absorb the ultraviolet rays. The darker the skin—even suntanned skin—the less ultraviolet light is absorbed. Therefore, black children are more susceptible to rickets, and they usually require supplementation.

Vitamin D destroyers

The skin has natural oils to maintain cellular integrity and health. These oils form a substance called 7-dehydrocholesterol. If a bath or shower is taken before or immediately after swimming and sun exposure, the oils are washed off and no vitamin D is absorbed.

Sun blocking creams also block the absorption of vitamin D. It is now known that more melanomas develop because of low vitamin D levels than from sunburns. Exposure to the sun a little each day and avoiding the sun at high noon are good measures to prevent sunburn. A certain combination of spice oils in extra virgin olive oil will stop the blistering, damage, and pain of sunburn by applying repeatedly every time the skin feels painful.

Infants and toddlers who suffer from rickets may not improve if they are thoroughly washed before sun exposure. If they do not seem to improve, it is better to wipe them with extra virgin olive oil rather than using soap and water.

There are common practices today that cause major destruction of this important vitamin. The residential water supplies are contaminated with the addition of fluorosilicic acid, a deadly byproduct of the aluminum industry. While this form of fluoride is added on the pretext that it is beneficial for the formation of healthy bones and teeth, there is ample evidence—solid proof—that this is a poison rather than a benefit. Further, it blocks the action of vitamin D for the prevention of rickets and other bone diseases. Plus, mineral oil should be avoided, since it prevents the absorption of vitamin D and the other fat soluble vitamins.

Vitamin D sources and requirements

Other than sunlight the best source of vitamin D has always been derived from fish liver oil such as cod liver oil or halibut liver oil. As mentioned earlier extensive refining may be the reason that the modern fish oils are not as effective as the old-time cod liver oil that many of our grandparents received.

The requirement of vitamin D is regulated and is now only 400 IUs. However, for years the infant requirement was 1000 units daily. Babies need sunlight exposure, as do mothers. Remember that soap and water can remove the oils on the skin that are converted to vitamin D by exposure to ultraviolet rays. Thus, bathing should be delayed until several hours after sun exposure. It once was a common practice that during at least the first month of life the infant was only given olive oil baths. It sounds like a rather "slippery" practice, but now we understand the reason. In England it is common to see the prams (baby buggies) in the parks on sunny days. The babies are covered but not so heavily that all sunlight is blocked. Unfortunately, in England there is a heavy amount of cloud cover, which blocks the ultraviolet rays. Since vitamin D is vital in the development of the child, once a day baby and mother must enjoy the benefits of the sun's rays for 10 to 30 minutes. If mother is nursing, four or more fish oil capsules (burbot or unfiltered Alaskan sockeye salmon oil) containing natural-source vitamin D are beneficial. Otherwise, fat soluble vitamins A and D are normally best absorbed with a meal containing fat from butter, cheese, milk, eggs, avocado, etc. While the recommended dosages of nutrients have been downsized to barely sustain life, most children can safely utilize natural vitamin D up to 1500 to 2000 units daily.

Many years ago Adelle Davis stated in her book *Let's Eat Right to Keep Fit* that a toxic dose of vitamin D for adults appeared to be 300,000 to 800,000 units per day. Needless to say, 400 IUs is a minimal dose and may not be enough to prevent bone deformity and other diseases. When large doses of vitamin D are required to cure and prevent any further damage due to rickets, additional intake of thiamine will protect against any adverse effects. Nutrients work together to make the body function well and to maintain good health.

The sunshine-derived vitamin D helps children to develop into strong and healthy adults. Their bone/skeletal formation, tooth development and structure, blood sugar/energy status, and eye health are dependent upon this most important vitamin. Once the bones harden, any damage, such as curvature of the spine, bowed legs, knock knees, jawbone deformities, and tooth misalignment, will be permanent. If a child has crooked teeth, don't just head to the orthodontist and believe that fate and bad luck caused the problem. Watch for the symptoms mentioned, and use sunshine and supplements to change the child's health for the better. Note: remember that bone damage and rickets usually occur during the infant/toddler stage. Again, damage may develop when growth spurts occur during the teen years. Be aware of deficiency signs, and refuse to use drugs or surgery when nutrition intervention is actually the only way to solve the problem. Otherwise the child's bone deformities are permanent. Even children whose families are blessed financially may suffer from these defects. Don't panic; just treat the child with plenty of good food and supplements, while under a caring doctor's supervision. Massage and other body work are also beneficial.

Vitamin E

In 1936 Evans and others were the first to derive vitamin E from wheat germ oil. However, in 1922 Evans and Bishop had already proved that it is essential for normal reproduction.

In 1931 researchers Goettsche and Pappernheimer determined that muscular dystrophy developed in guinea pigs and rabbits which were deprived of vitamin E. Children who had this dreaded disease took vitamin E with some success.

While alpha tocopherol has long been touted as the most desirable form of vitamin E, the mixed tocopherols—alpha, beta, gamma, delta, and three other tocopherols as found in foods—are, certainly, beneficial for the body. Little to no research has been done to determine the exact action of the other tocopherols in relation to alpha tocopherol. Yet, the combination as found in nature is surely ideal for the body's needs. Naturally occurring vitamins plus their known and unknown co-factors are why rich, organic food sources of vitamins are always the best choices.

How vitamin E functions in the body

Vitamin E is a fat soluble vitamin, and more E is found in the healthy body than any other vitamin. It is needed for muscular health as demonstrated by the increase of muscular dystrophy in children with low vitamin E levels. Also, the heart is a very important organ requiring vitamin E, and it is a muscle. Vitamin E is an important antioxidant, so it keeps fat from becoming rancid and helps the body to use fat appropriately. It also protects vitamin A, linoleic acid, and other nutrients, such as B complex and biotin, from the toxicity of rancid fats and oxidation in the body. The main concentration of vitamin E is in the pituitary, adrenals, and the sex glands. Nevertheless, the significance of this vitamin for bodily functions is still not totally understood. Yet, it is known that anyone with an overactive thyroid gland requires more than the normal daily allowance. The brain and central nervous system are also protected by this essential vitamin.

In premature babies deficiency in vitamin E may cause retinal damage. Unfortunately, they are usually fed synthetic formulas which may be low in vitamin E. Also, if the mother had a low level during gestation, the tiny infant will have none stored. If this is not corrected, blindness may result. A premature baby thrives much better on mother's expressed breast milk and her loving touch whenever possible. All nursing mothers should be certain to have generous amounts of vitamin E in their diets, especially those who contribute breast milk for the premature babies.

Other deficiency symptoms in children include problems with walking and coordination, abnormal reflexes, frequent falling, abnormal red blood cells, heart abnormalities, fragile capillaries, incomplete digestion of fats, and scarring of wounds. There are also toxic reactions due to mercury, lead, nitrates and nitrites, as well as other noxious chemicals and food additives. A weak immune system is also notable with a vitamin E deficit. Certainly, cancer is on the increase in children. It is important to be aware that research studies conducted with rats showed that cancer tissue did not grow when the blood serum was enriched with vitamin E. However, it did grow readily in serum lacking this vitamin.

Vitamin E sources and requirements

Good sources of natural vitamin E are limited. It is available in small amounts in nuts, seeds, egg yolk, carrots, tomatoes, lettuce and other dark green leafy vegetables, and whole grains. Wheat germ oil is a good source, but many children are allergic to wheat. Freshly ground whole meal flour and unprocessed cereals are usually dependable sources of vitamin E. Commercial vegetable oils are so processed that most if not all of the vitamin E is destroyed. Cold-pressed organic sesame oil is a rich source. Sesame seed oil is easily added to dressings, shakes, and many other recipes. Black seed oil and Austrian pumpkinseed oil also contain vitamin E if they are cold-pressed premium-grade oils. They all should be added at the end of cooking or poured over food like a sauce at the table. They should not be used in cooking and baking or for frying.

Other foods that contain little or no vitamin E are butter, cream, dried and pasteurized milk, fruits, yeast, lard, fish liver oils, polished rice, white flour, and refined cornmeal.

Note: Most cornmeal is genetically modified with viral vectors. These are used to transport the genetic material from certain bacteria. These bacterial genes code (send out messages) for the production of pesticides. Therefore, when you eat genetically engineered corn, you are eating man-made pesticides. It is unfit for human consumption, because it contains animal parts which are placed within natural vegetation. This completely disrupts the human immune system, leading to a wide range of toxic reactions. Ultimately, it can increase the risks for serious diseases such as heart disease, diabetes, and cancer. Unfortunately, cross pollenization is causing contamination of the organic corn as well. There will soon be little to no corn on earth that is fit to consume thanks to genetic engineering.

While natural food is best, most food is so nutritionally depleted that it is inadequate. Children need 200 IU to 800 IU of vitamin E daily depending upon the health status. Kodak makes most of the vitamin E commonly found in health food stores. It is derived from soy, but unfortunately, that means it is corrupted with genetically modified organisms. This may be hazardous to a child's life. Using the suggested foods and oils on a daily basis will solve the vitamin E requirement most of the time. Fortunately, there is a supplement option. Organic sunflower sources of vitamin E are limited, but they are available. This supplement form is an extract of sunflower seed oil, providing all the various types of natural vitamin E. While supplies are limited, check with superior health stores for this purely natural vitamin E complex.

Vitamin K

Vitamin K, named after the word koagulation, is in the fat soluble family. In 1931 McFarlane noted that chickens, when fed fish meal, were cured of hemorrhagic disease. When they were given fish meal which had the fat extracted, there was no benefit.

Vitamin K causes blood to clot. However, it will not stop hemorrhage. Hemophilia, a bleeding disease which occurs in males, does not respond to vitamin K treatment.

How vitamin K works in the body

Only a small amount of vitamin K is stored in the liver. There, it mainly functions as a co-enzyme, which helps in the formation of a water soluble protein called prothrombin. Prothrombin is an important substance in the blood plasma which is involved in the blood clotting mechanism.

No one really knows all the functions of vitamin K. However, recent research shows that it may have an effect on behavior and bone disorders.

Vitamin K sources and requirements

Vitamin K is plentiful in burbot liver oil, alfalfa, and spinach. Good sources are green cabbage, cauliflower, kale, seaweed, tomatoes, liver, lean meat, egg yolk, and strawberries. Use organic or wild foods only, whenever possible.

Besides the plant and animal sources, vitamin K is produced by bacteria in the large intestine. If the intestinal flora is healthy, there should be no reason for a deficiency. The sources of vitamin K mentioned above are safe and are readily and appropriately utilized in the body. Synthetic vitamin K, which is only available through prescription, is the only type which may be toxic.

Dietary requirements are not really certain for vitamin K. However, deficiencies are reported. Because the flora is not firmly established in the infant, hospitals administer vitamin K to the mother just before birth. This is because the infant's prothrombin levels decrease and do not normalize until around the beginning of the second week.

Even a minor accidental injury could cause the newborn to hemorrhage while the vitamin K level is low. Brain hemorrhage could occur, which would cause spastic paralysis. Then, the resulting loss of muscular control and jerky movements would be a permanent handicap.

There are other factors which increase the need for vitamin K. A rise in body temperature may increase the need for vitamin K. Also, aspirin and other drugs may cause a deficiency due to diarrhea or liver damage. (Never use aspirin when a child has a fever. Reye's Syndrome could result.)

Vitamin K is important as a clotting factor for all ages. It is also a necessary component in building bone tissue. Intestinal bacteria is the most important means of producing vitamin K, so probiotics may be beneficial. Dark green leafy vegetables and alfalfa meal are excellent sources, but the most dense source is fermented burbot liver oil. There is no established requirement for this vitamin.

Essential fatty acids

Omega-3 and -6

Some people believe that little to no fat should be eaten. Yet, the essential fatty acids are vital to maintain the health and development of a child. The first signs of deficiency are failure to thrive and gain weight, dry scaly skin, scaling behind the ears, infantile eczema, dandruff, acne, boils, and diarrhea. Then, the immune system is affected. Colds and flu occur more often. Soon, other signs develop, such as dry brittle hair and nails, falling hair, asthma, impaired retinal development—especially in infants, and kidney disease.

The essential oils are also important as a support system. They combine with vitamin D in making calcium available to the tissues. This is done by aiding in the assimilation of phosphorus and by nourishing the skin. Also these important oils are necessary for the function and maintenance of the adrenal glands and the thyroid gland.

If a child is deficient in the essential fatty acids for a prolonged time, he/she will likely develop abnormal deposits on the inside walls of the blood vessels. The wrong fats in the diet can cause circulatory conditions and hardening of the arteries even at an early age. Always remember, all margarine should have a hazardous chemical warning on it. This is because of the harmful trans fatty acids from hydrogenated oils. All refined oils and hydrogenated oils should never be consumed. Besides poisoning the system, they also compete for absorption with the important essential fatty acid.

The omega-3 oil research shows that since the brain is composed of mostly fat, the essential fatty acids help the brain to develop. Children seem to learn faster and easier. Not only does learning improve, but also the children are much more attentive and cooperative.

Like the omega-3 fatty acids, omega-6 fatty acids have certain functions and benefits. Both of them are needed to reduce the development and incidence of heart disease, cancer, and diabetes even among the very young. The omega-6 fatty acid as gamma linoleic acid (GLA) has anti-inflammatory benefits. It also contributes to weight loss by activating the metabolism and increasing the caloric burn. GLA has proven to be helpful in decreasing hyperactivity in children. Since omega-3 and -6 fatty acids are known to benefit brain development and behavior, wouldn't supplementation with essential fatty acids be far more logical and desirable than giving children mind-altering drugs?

Omega-3 and -6 sources and requirements

Omega-3 is commonly found as EPA or eicosapentaenoic acid and DHA or docosahexaenoic acid in cold-water fish. While it is beneficial, the oceans are continuously poisoned with contamination from every conceivable source that our "civilized" world can produce. The common more dangerous toxins are methylmercury, dioxin, and polychlorinated biphenyls. As mentioned repeatedly, most fish oils are super refined in an effort to eliminate those and many other dangerous toxins. Likewise, beneficial substances are removed in the refining process, and the processing itself is questionable.

The remarkable substances in cold-water fish oils work together to eliminate pain, illness, and deficiency symptoms. For troubled children it is a God-send. Many reports and studies show good results for children with attention deficit and learning disorders. All children benefit from good fish oils in some way. Vision improvements have been regularly noted. It is especially beneficial for brain development and memory enhancement. Fish oils are available in capsules and are a good source of EPA. Even cod liver oil capsules contain a small amount of EPA. However, wild Alaskan sockeye salmon oil is an excellent source of the more absorbable triglyceride forms of omega-3s. This includes EPA, DHA, and the important companion fatty acids. Vitamins A and D as well as astaxanthin, a beautiful bright coral-colored carotenoid and antioxidant more powerful than vitamin E, are also components in the unfiltered sockeye salmon oil. This source is as pristine as is possible to find on this planet. This cold-water fish oil contains all the cofactors that are usually lost in processing. It saved the life of a critically ill Beluga whale. Her two whales friends were also ill. The sockeye salmon oil did not arrive in time for them. Sadly, they did not survive. Another significant response occurred with a polar bear in a zoo. The keepers spread the oil on the wall of the bear's compound. He walked away from a meat meal to lick the wall clean of the sockeye salmon oil. Animals instinctively know what is nutritionally beneficial for them. Humans did too at one time, but it is a fairly rare occurrence today.

Austrian pumpkinseed oil made from cold-pressed seeds of the Styrian pumpkin is another excellent source of the omega fatty acids. This oil tastes so good and can be put into shakes, over salads, baked potatoes and sweet potatoes, and in tomato juice. It is much tastier than many nut and seed oils and does not oxidize like flaxseed oil. Flaxseed oil can even become rancid inside the body after consumption, especially for those with digestive issues. The Austrians use the cold-pressed pumpkinseed oil daily as a condiment on their food. Give small children one teaspoon and older children and teenagers from one to two tablespoons of the best quality, cold-pressed pumpkinseed seed oil each day. It is also possible to rotate with other fine sources of essential fatty acids. Small children need around 5 drops a day and for older children up to a dropperful of essential fatty acids is beneficial. Essential fatty acids are also derived from the seeds of berries. This is a highly nutritious, safe source and quite tasty too. Quality is always of utmost importance when selecting any oil.

The omega-6 fatty acids and some GLA are available in evening primrose oil, borage oil, black raspberry seed oil, and black currant seed oil. More importantly, GLA is in human milk. That is the main clue how very necessary this substance is. The berry seed oils in the morning smoothie or other foods such as hot cereal and milk will add a lovely flavor and intense nourishment.

The essential fatty acids are needed for brain development, adrenal and thyroid functioning, skin health, cholesterol and hormone balance, protection from many diseases, and anti-inflammatory properties. Everyone needs them.

Children who rarely consume essential fatty acids are deprived. It does not matter if they are from the poorest or richest families in the world. Once you learn to recognize the deficiency symptoms, it is shocking how common they are. When children suffer these defects, it is not their fault. Parents and adults in responsible positions where children are congregated must become aware of how to identify the deficiencies and how to eliminate them. I see children who have difficulties learning and remembering. Then there are those with dry, scaling skin and dermatitis. Many children today suffer from asthma, allergies, immune disorders, and even heart disease, arthritis, and cancer. The essential fatty acids protect the cells and keep the cell walls soft and pliable. Thus, they are able to ward off viruses, bacteria, carcinogens, and allergens. But the essential fatty acids must always be available in their bodies to achieve this feat. For those who consume the Standard American Diet, there is no hope that they are getting the essential fatty acids that they so direly need. Again, kids need care. Let's give them the fuel that they need to be the best that they can be. Keep in mind that what is done to build up an individual physically as a child is the health foundation for that person for the rest of adulthood.

MINERALS

Minerals are vital for life, and they are often described as the spark plugs of the body. They are the enzymatic activators, and many of them combine to form the skeletal structure of the body. Life could not exist without the minerals. Furthermore, vitamins without minerals are virtually worthless.

In the 1960s Carlson Wade reported that the government understood the importance of minerals for learning and cognition. Senate Document 264 revealed that mineral-deficient mice were unable to navigate a maze. However, the mice well-nourished with minerals were quickly able to find their way through it. Further and even more frightening is the fact that disease conditions in mice can be caused or curtailed "by controlling only the minerals in their food."

Today, virtually 100 percent of all people in the United States are mineral deficient. The mineral content of the American food supply decreases yearly. Factory farming has caused this dearth in food that is supposed to nourish the body. This severe deficiency is a major cause of sudden death in children. Likewise, the high incidence of childhood obesity continues to grow. Also, too many children in this nation are plagued with massive behavioral problems and learning difficulties, and the numbers continue to increase. Today in Chicago alone obesity among third graders is at 39 percent. All of this is correlated to mineral deficit.

It is common that children are given mind-altering drugs if they are disruptive in any way. Never is it commonly the first choice to alter the diet and lifestyles of these children. Irritable, quarrelsome children can become balanced and friendly. They will sleep better just by fortifying the diet with calcium. The so-called "stupid" or slow, backward type behavior is typically due to severe deficiencies in magnesium and other important nutrients. When these deficiencies are addressed, the results are amazing. For a truly vibrant and healthy child it also means altering the diet for the better. This means the sugar, chemicals and food dyes, GMOs, poor quality food, and the junk in general must be deleted as a commonly accepted way of life.

The following true story is an example of how children are dealt with in today's society instead of requiring what they really need, which is supplementation and dietary improvements. I was counseling a middle-income mother, who had five children. Her youngest child was a beautiful little blue-eyed blonde boy, who could not sit down. He always had a smile on his little face, but he was constantly moving and into everything. It also was determined that he had a certain unpleasant body odor even immediately after a bath. This little fellow was about to enter kindergarten. At the pre-registration interview Mom had been warned that he would be put on Ritalin or expelled if she was unable to alter his behavior. Because of the incessant activity and the body odor (five-year-old children are not supposed to stink), I knew he was deficient in minerals and vitamins. Thus, his mother was advised to give him an easy-to-take calcium, magnesium, and zinc supplement.

Every day she gave him the liquid form of these minerals. She stated that he soon calmed down and smelled better too. A few months later I asked if she was continuing the minerals. Her answer was no. That absolutely shocked me. I asked why she would discontinue them, since he was doing so well. She said he loved the liquid minerals too much and went through a bottle in less than a week The cost of the minerals was a whopping $6.00 a bottle, and yet, he could have all the pop and junk food he wanted. Furthermore, she stated that the Ritalin was free, and the school would not allow the child to take minerals. He could take Ritalin at school, but he was not allowed to take anything nourishing. She said it was just too much trouble to fight the system. Note: when such a direly mineral-deficient child is fully repleted with the minerals that he/she needs, the craving for the liquid minerals diminishes accordingly. Thought for the day: how can a mind-altering drug fulfill the need for missing nutrients? However, it must not matter as long as the school gets a kickback for every child placed and kept on drugs throughout his/her school experience. Also keep in mind that the perpetrators of every school massacre have been on or just come off of mind-altering drugs.

ESSENTIAL MACRO-MINERALS THAT KIDS NEED MOST

Calcium

Calcium is usually the first and, perhaps, the only one that people recall when asked to mention the name of a mineral. It is commonly discussed on television, and even the orange juice companies are fortifying the juice with it. It is fairly well understood that it is a basic component of the skeletal system and teeth. While there is only a tiny amount in the blood and tissues, calcium is needed for vital life support functions such as the normal contraction and relaxation (the latter being due to magnesium) of muscles, especially the heart, for the blood clotting mechanism, for the appropriate transport of body fluids through the cell walls, normal blood pressure, for the sensitive acid-alkaline balance in the body, and for nerve impulse transmission and central nervous system regulation.

When children are nervous and irritable, their blood calcium levels are, undoubtedly, low. Frequently, behavioral difficulties are significantly decreased when calcium is increased in the diet. To provide added sources of calcium children should have snacks of something like the following: lightly steamed "trees" (broccoli) with real cheese sauce, soaked almonds, almond butter on a celery stick, cheese and almond butter in a collard leaf roll-up, or goat's milk and yogurt smoothies. Full-fat milk, yogurt, and cheese must always be used to protect the intestinal walls from the milk sugar known as galactose. Galactose in skim milk causes irritation of the bowel walls. The constant use of skim milk causes inflammation of the bowels and may even lead to cancer. Also, the fat soluble vitamins A and D (fat must be present for those vitamins to be absorbed) plus vitamin C and phosphorus are necessary for calcium to be absorbed and properly utilized.

Children grow at different rates. Some have growth spurts, where they seem to shoot up inches over night. A diet rich in calcium and other nutrients is required from infancy through the teen years to support their development into strong and healthy adults. Healthy food is important to build healthy bones. Height is an indicator of mineral sufficiency. Yet, to maintain the blood calcium levels, the body will take what it needs directly from the bones, usually the spine and the pelvis. Thus, children who mainly eat deficient, processed foods and fast foods, as well as large amounts of sugar in all forms, are more likely to have shorter stature than those who avoid these. They are also more likely to easily break bones, or be afflicted with scoliosis, dental caries, heart abnormalities, blood sugar irregularities, and other diseases.

Phosphorus

Phosphorus must be in a proper ratio with calcium to be appropriately utilized in the body, and that ratio is 2 parts calcium to 1 part phosphorus. Vitamin D plays a significant role in regulating the balance of these two minerals. Sunshine is very important for the production of vitamin D, but perhaps fortified milk, fish liver oil, and maca, the latter being a Peruvian root vegetable, are more reliable sources during the winter months.

Like calcium most of the phosphorus is found in the bones and the teeth. The remainder, about 20 to 30 percent, vies with magnesium as being the most active mineral in the body. Moreover, it is found in every cell. It is necessary for activating the power in cellular metabolism. Phosphorus combines with alkaline substances to keep the blood relatively neutral. For mental acuity phosphorus is needed in the production of cerebrin and lecithin.

Carbohydrates, proteins, and fats can not be properly synthesized and utilized in the body without phosphorus. While it is needed for the processes of muscle contraction, nerve activity, kidney function, and some hormonal secretions, it also transports substances, such as the fatty acids, to locations throughout the body for immediate use or storage. Since phosphorus plays such an important role in fat and starch metabolism, its deficiency may be a component in some cases of obesity.

Mentation (thought processes) and brain functions are constantly developing during childhood, especially during the first five years of life. The brain is mostly composed of liquid, and the remaining solid mass is phosphorized fats. As growth of the nervous system and, thus, the capacity for wisdom increases, the fat mass also increases. Thus, putting a child on a low-fat diet causes a deficiency in both fat soluble vitamins and phosphorized fats for brain development. Children should be fed good fats such as cold-pressed extra virgin olive oil, Styrian pumpkinseed oil, sesame oil, coconut oil, palm oil, butter, and full-fat dairy products. Never feed them margarine, refined cooking oils, and solid hydrogenated or partially hydrogenated fats, and that also means no fried foods cooked in these dangerous fats. That actually eliminates most all fast foods and packaged, prepared, fried foods. This includes potato chips, as well as frozen fried foods which are warmed in the oven such as fish sticks, chicken fingers, and French fries.

Since phosphorus is so important in the body, this raises the question is it necessary to supplement the diet with it? Usually, this mineral is plentiful in fresh foods. It is largely found in protein foods. It is also abundant in soda pop drinks as phosphoric acid. However, this phosphoric acid is not desirable, and soda pop drinks are also loaded with sugar, which adversely affects the delicate calcium/phosphorus balance in the body. The best choices for drinks are purified and mineral water, herbal teas, and freshly made juices.

Magnesium

Magnesium is also essential for the skeletal structure, the teeth, and the cells of the body. It acts as a catalyst for the enzymes that release energy from glucose (blood sugar), and it activates or inactivates many additional enzyme systems. This is why it is such a necessary component for liver cells.

Irritability and extreme nervousness with over reaction to sounds and any kind of disturbance are good indicators of magnesium deficit. ADD/ADHD anyone? This is certainly a relevant factor, since magnesium is a relaxant. It helps an individual to maintain a calm composure even under stress. Furthermore, it acts as a coolant, helping to prevent the ill effects of hot weather. For sleep problems a magnesium-rich diet is important. However, a magnesium supplement should not be used just before bedtime, since it can then act as an energizer.

Deficiency symptoms are easy to recognize. Nervous twitches and tremors are common signs of deficiency. Most children who are deficient have failure to thrive, and they have little appetite. A rapid heartbeat, confusion and disorientation, as well as nausea and vomiting, occur when magnesium levels are too low. Calcium deposits also develop as a result of the deficiency.

Muscle tissues (cells) require magnesium, and severe cramping results when there is a deficiency. Severe muscle cramping usually in the legs and feet can be relieved with magnesium-rich food and supplementation. Magnesium relieves severe muscle contractions and relaxes the nerve impulses, while calcium stimulates them.

The only reliable laboratory test to determine magnesium status is called the red blood cell magnesium test. It shows how much of this mineral is inside the red blood cell, while the magnesium in the blood alone is not a true indicator. Even superior to this is symptom and sign testing, as found in *Nutrition Tests for Better Health,* by Dr. Cass Ingram (Knowledge House Publishers). This is because symptoms and signs are an established record of the body functions and its needs.

Anyone who has diarrhea and vomiting for a prolonged time is magnesium deficient. Also, drinking distilled or reverse osmosis water on a daily basis will eventually cause a deficiency. The red blood cell test determines the degree of deficiency. If the level is dangerously low, a physician may need to give a magnesium push (IV), since taking supplements in high doses has a laxative effect.

Magnesium-rich foods are the most desirable source of this mineral. A raw vegetable- and enzyme-rich fruit juice drink made from organic beet greens, kale, carrots, pineapple juice, and powdered sunflower seeds will provide a delicious magnesium boost. Fresh raw organic foods are always best, because for maximum absorption of magnesium, other nutrients such as calcium, phosphorus, protein, and vitamin D must also be adequately available. It is believed that a desirable calcium/magnesium ratio is two parts calcium to one part magnesium. However, research continues to reveal the importance and need for magnesium throughout the body.

Other good food sources include organic figs, lemons, grapefruits, almonds and other oil-rich nuts and seeds, wild rice, apples, celery, leafy vegetables, oregano, whole grain cereals, and milk. The more that foods are processed and refined, the more the mineral content will be adversely affected. One of the top sources is the germ of grains and seeds, especially rice bran and germ. One combination made from crushed rice bran, rice germ, fortified flax, and red sour grape is the ideal whole food magnesium supplement, containing some 20 percent of the RDA in three tablespoons.

Infants require 50 to 70 mg of magnesium daily. Young children should have around 150 mg of the mineral in their diets daily, and older children need around 250 mg. Teens require 300 to 400 mg daily. These amounts vary according to size, activity, and state of health.

Potassium

Potassium must be in balance with sodium, since sodium regulates the fluids outside the cells, and potassium is basically within the cells. These minerals, known as electrolytes, help keep the heartbeat stable as well as nourish all muscles in the body.

Potassium has countless functions. The brain needs a constant oxygen supply. The minerals potassium and phosphorus unite to provide this oxygen source. The kidneys need potassium, since it activates them to remove any waste material. Without an adequate supply of this vital mineral the kidneys may enlarge and the bones may be brittle. Likewise, a deficiency in the blood can cause symptoms such as digestive disturbances, constipation, heartbeat abnormalities, muscle damage, sleep disturbances, and nervous upset. Potassium in the cell is needed for the metabolism of carbohydrates and proteins.

Children should enjoy citrus fruits as a good source of potassium, unless they are allergic to them. Figs, avocado, green peppers, bananas, mint tea, and most vegetables and fruit are good sources. Beans and lentils are good sources, but they are difficult for children to digest.

Sodium and Chloride

Sodium and chloride are commonly combined as sodium chloride salts. Without chloride the body could not make hydrochloric acid in the stomach. Hydrochloric acid is needed for digestion of food, especially the protein foods. Sodium and chloride are part of the electrolyte system that must be in balance with potassium. Too much sodium causes fluid retention. As well, too much or too little sodium affects the acid-base balance of the body. Sodium is also necessary for proper nerve and muscle function. Any child who has weak adrenal glands—the body's coping mechanisms—will need extra sodium. Sea salt is a desirable source. If a child seems to crave salt, it should not be restricted or withheld. One couple had a child who wanted salt on everything. The doctor told them to restrict the child's sodium intake. He had severe adrenal weakness and direly needed the extra sodium. The small boy repeatedly climbed into the cupboards to eat salt. They couldn't keep him away from the salt, so they took it totally out of the home. Sadly, the child died due to the forced sodium deprivation. Obviously, he was following his natural instincts. Repetitive instinctual behavior should be observed and respected. Only consult with doctors who are wise enough to do what is correct for the child. Sea salt contains many minerals. Good brands with no contaminants are perfectly safe and a good source of trace minerals.

Sodium chloride (chlorine) acts as a blood and lymph cleanser. This is because sodium chloride helps to keep other minerals in a soluble state so they do not clog and harden throughout the circulatory system. Sodium also helps keep calcium in suspension in the blood. This is necessary for strong and healthy nerves and a happy, calm child.

Chlorine also helps the liver to filter out toxic material. It is a valuable component for healthy joints and ligaments. It is also needed for driving the endocrine hormones to the sites that need them.

If your child seems to have problems digesting and has weight loss and gas, it may be due to sodium deficiency. (Note: it may also be a sign of parasite infestation.) Along with those symptoms if the muscles seem to be flaccid or shrinking do consider sodium depletion.

Sodium is an important element for all the digestive juices and enzymes. It is required for the secretion of digestive salts and intestinal fluids. The process is quite complex. When these important substances are disrupted, the digestion of fats, carbohydrates, and amino acids is also disrupted. This leads to malabsorption of nutrients.

Dandelion greens are an excellent source of natural sodium. Make a big salad or juice the greens with carrots and beets. For natural chloride sources use green leafy vegetables, kelp, dulse and other sea vegetables, ripe olives, and rye flour. It is obviously not the same as the chemical chlorine added to municipal water systems, which is hazardous to health.

Common table salt is not a desirable source of sodium chloride. It is heated and processed. Plus, various flowing agents and chemicals which contain aluminum are added. Even a form of sugar known as dextrose is combined with the salt. A good sea salt is a better choice.

Sulfur

Sulfur is an important part of all protein-containing foods. It is a component of B_1 (thiamine), biotin, and certain amino acids such as methionine and cysteine. It is part of the structure of every cell of the body, and it works with the mineral salts to maintain the acid-base balance in the body.

While thiamine helps in the release of energy from glucose, sulfur is needed in the production of insulin. Glutathione and other metabolic regulators also need sulfur in their makeup.

There is no daily requirement for sulfur, since it is found abundantly in all protein foods. However, vegans and even vegetarians who are not getting animal protein could potentially be deficient. Low sulfur levels may cause sluggishness and chronic tiredness. Collagen formation, tissue building, and respiration are dependent on adequate amounts of sulfur. That means skin integrity and growth of the child would be affected with low protein intake and, thus, low sulfur intake. Too much sulfur, of course, is toxic. Natural food sources of sulfur include eggs, fish, lean beef, organ meats, cabbage, beans, and Brussels sprouts.

ESSENTIAL TRACE MINERALS FOR PERFECT HEALTH

Trace minerals are needed for metabolic processes. They are also required for transport activity. However, only tiny amounts are actually used by the body. The research on how these trace minerals function is ongoing. So many are found in the body, and yet, researchers still have no idea why most of them are present and what purposes they serve. Food processing destroys or inactivates 70 to 90 percent of the essential and trace minerals. The only reason for this processing is to extend the shelf life of the product. When people are deficient in these substances, and possibly 100 percent of all humans are, it is impossible to enjoy the perfect health that God meant for us to have.

As will be shown, even though the amounts are small, these trace minerals are extraordinary in their importance. Without them the body is at risk for the development of a wide range of diseases or may even fail to survive.

William Quesnell proved that minerals are more important than vitamins in human nutrition. He stated that the body can use minerals without vitamins, but vitamins are useless without minerals. All minerals are important in their particular function and realm. The quantity of a mineral found in the body does not make it the most important. In other words even though calcium and magnesium are the two most plentiful minerals in the body, other minerals are needed to complete their particular activities. The proper balance of all minerals is the real determining factor in relation to health.

When you purchase food, the source is most important. For example, grapes grown in Europe can sustain life even as a single food source. In other words, if that was the only food available, a person eating them, including the seeds, could survive and actually thrive. This is not so with American grapes. Plus, much of the American grape production are hybrids, which are seedless. They do not have the same mineral and overall nutrient content. Thus, they are inadequate as a complete food source. Grapes from two different locations may look the same, but one source may be deficient in minerals such as chromium and cobalt. Yet, the price for the nutrient-dense food may be the same as the nutrient-depleted one.

The mineral content affects the amount of other nutrients found in food. For example, nutrients, such as vitamin C, beta carotene, and even amino acids, are dependent on the presence of certain minerals. The following charts represent the benefits of optimum levels and problems caused by deficiencies of the trace minerals. The following are a few examples that show the immense role minerals play in plant nutrition and, therefore, in the nutrient content of foods.

Mineral: optimum level increases nutrient content

copper	vitamin C in barley; carotene in barley, wheat, oats, spinach and carrots
boron	tryptophan in alfalfa (tryptophan can be converted to niacin in the body, if needed)
manganese	carotene in vegetation

Mineral deficiencies cause the following:

molybdenum	decreased vitamin C in tomatoes and other vegetables
cobalt	B_{12} cannot be produced; results in excess absorption of aluminum from fruit, nuts, grains, and vegetables
cesium	results in excess absorption of aluminum from fruit, nuts, grains, and vegetables

Today, refined food is virtually devoid of minerals. Yet, even organic foods will not be replete with minerals if the soil is depleted. About 60 percent of the topsoil in the United States has been destroyed, and poor farming practices account for much of this. In many countries throughout the world the topsoil is about one foot deep and rich in mineral matter. In the United States the top soil is around five to six inches deep with little remaining trace minerals. This depleted soil bears depleted food.

There are over 70 minerals present in healthy blood. The blood circulates the minerals and nutrients throughout the body. It deposits these life-giving components, wherever they are needed. All 70 minerals are not explained in this book, because many have not been researched. Thus, no one knows their purpose. Likewise, even with those that have been researched, the full extent of their true importance remains unknown.

The essential trace minerals are necessary for good health and energy. The information in this next section represents what research currently reports as accepted knowledge.

Iodine

Discovered around 5000 years ago, iodine is claimed to be the oldest known essential trace mineral. At that time this unknown factor in seaweed helped to prevent the enlargement of the thyroid gland. This swelling of the thyroid gland in the neck is called goiter.

Iodine is utilized by the thyroid to make the hormone thyroxin. This hormone is composed of approximately 65 percent iodine. Thyroxin is needed for maintaining body temperature and the basal metabolic rate. The metabolic rate governs how fast fuel is burned in the body due to oxygen content. It is also necessary in the regulation of growth and development of every individual.

When infants are deficient in thyroid hormones, they develop cretinism. Usually, even before birth there is a lack of iodine. They do not develop appropriately either physically or mentally. Both failure to thrive physically and severe mental retardation may result just because of a lack of this single mineral.

Yet, it is so easy to obtain this mineral. It is readily available in sea foods, seaweed, and other saltwater plants such as dulse. Iodized salt is a source of iodine. However, iodized sea salt is preferable. This is because table salt contains dextrose, a sugar derived from genetically engineered corn. Aluminum, which is an anti-caking/flowing agent, is another common additive. Sea salt does not contain iodine unless it is fortified. There is an Antarctic-source sea salt plus seaweed in small flakes in a salt grinder. It is especially tasty and fulfills the need for iodine nicely. Wild, raw salt capsules, fortified with crushed wild kelp and oregano, are also available as an easy way to get the minimum need for salt and iodine. Both are available at www.Americanwildfoods.com.

Processed food is rarely seasoned with iodized salt, and this is unfortunate. There is as much iodine in food as is available in the soil, where it is grown. Many times, this means there is little to no iodine for nourishment. Then, even when there is a trace of iodine, it is lost during manufacturing processes. So, that is why iodized salt is preferable for manufactured food. A few people are allergic to iodine, so it should be noted on the label.

Salt got its bad reputation from the highly refined, adulterated substance which is commonly known as table salt. The delicate balance of trace minerals is damaged in the processing by using high heat to dry it. Then, by adding sugar, aluminum, and other chemicals, it is made even less desirable.

Inland areas worldwide have little to no iodine in the soil. Thus, many Canadians suffer the consequences from a lack of this mineral, which are goiter and thyroid gland inflammation. The usual treatments are to remove the swollen thyroid or destroy this gland with radioactive iodine. The suffering of these hypothyroid victims is compounded by such radical actions.

In countries where kelp and dulse are commonly eaten few have thyroid problems. These sea plants provide a huge amount of minerals, including iodine. These plants are constantly in seawater, so pollution is a major consideration. Everyone should find the cleanest possible sources and use these sea plants on a weekly basis. Some use dulse and certain delicate seaweeds as a crunchy, salty snack. These seaweeds can also be soaked in water to soften the dried plants and to remove some of the salt. Then, they can be cut into pieces and used in soups, salads, with whole grain or rice pasta, or even on sandwiches.

Iron

Iron makes up the oxygen-transporting proteins in the body. In the blood this is called hemoglobin. This substance is the carrier of oxygen which makes the red blood cells red in color. Myoglobin causes oxygen to stay in the muscles for quick access when needed. Oxygen is so important that there can be no life without it.

Hemoglobin carries carbon dioxide from the cells to the lungs where the CO_2 is then exhaled from the body. Then, oxygen is again picked up in the lungs and carried to the cells for energy production throughout the body.

When the iron level is low, there are several symptoms. First, the child will be pale, tired, and anemic. Doctors look at the nails and the inside of the lower eyelids to determine the degree of anemia before testing. When anemia is a problem, muscle function is impaired and physical activity is difficult. Brain work is also impacted, and the anemic child may be a slow learner. He/she may also be easily distracted, cannot focus on lessons, and is slow to develop normal physical and mental skills. In some cases the child may complain of feeling cold or stand next to heat registers. He/she is seemingly susceptible to every immune challenge, and even wound healing will be more pronounced and take longer than usual.

When iron is plentiful in the body, it is stored in the liver, spleen, and bone marrow. As the red blood cells wear out, the stored iron is used to make new cells. A deficiency of iron in children may be a sign of malnutrition. However, it may also be a sign of intestinal parasites.

For best absorption and use throughout the body iron must be taken with B_{12}, folic acid, and vitamin C. It should also be taken with calcium, cobalt, copper, and phosphorus. In addition, hydrochloric acid in the stomach is necessary for its assimilation as well as the assimilation of calcium. Sometimes, there is little to no hydrochloric acid available, especially in those who consume a vegan diet. Those necessary hydrogen ions are sourced from protein foods such as seafood, fish, meat, dairy products, and eggs.

The food preservative EDTA, aspirin, antacids, and vitamin E are iron antagonists. That means the iron cannot be effectively utilized if taken with these substances. With the exception of vitamin E, children should avoid the above mentioned substances. Vitamin E supplements should always be consumed at a different time than iron supplements. It is a questionable practice when vitamin E and iron are combined in a multiple vitamin pill.

Some of the best food sources of iron are from organic meat, especially organic liver and organic eggs from free-range chickens. Iron from those sources is readily used by the body, if hydrochloric acid is present in the stomach. Dark leafy greens, which are rich in vitamin C, are good sources. Dark green vegetables are good natural sources of iron as well. So is maca. Grains and cereals usually provide a certain amount of iron, but the phytates and gluten can be a problem. The gluten can actually destroy the intestinal wall, leading to malabsorption. Other natural sources of iron include molasses (grape, carob, date, and pomegranate), raisins, apricots, and peaches. Too much iron is a risk factor as well, since it can be stored. Therefore, skip the synthetic supplements and, thus, the possibility of toxic overload. The daily dietary recommendations for infants are 10 to 15 mg; for children the range is 15 to 18 mg; for teens especially girls and active boys around 18 mg is usually appropriate.

Chromium

Chromium has only recently been recognized for its importance as a glucose tolerance factor. This is important for the utilization of insulin in the body and the regulation of blood sugar. Other research shows that it is beneficial for increasing the good HDL cholesterol.

Children who are raised on the Standard American Diet and junk food suffer from the consequences of chromium deficiency. A male child I know was fed fast food meals on a daily basis. I told his family that it was just a matter of time before he would be wearing glasses. Unfortunately, the prediction soon came true. When there is a lack of chromium and the diet is high in starch and sugar, the eyes are damaged. This causes myopia, which is also known as nearsightedness. Likewise, his stature and overall growth have been affected, and he is obese. Chromium is needed for the synthesis of essential fatty acids, cholesterol, and protein. With such a lack of nutrients throughout the boy's life, his whole digestive system has severely degenerated. He has a serious condition known as mega colon. Mega colon means that the bowel has no tone and has been severely stretched by constant constipation from eating food devoid of nourishment and fiber.

In this condition the contents of the bowel are extremely difficult to eliminate. It should be no surprise that he is a slow learner and a prime candidate for atherosclerosis as well as diabetes. Sadly, this is a true story. The boy has just recently become a teenager, so his bad eating habits are firmly established, as are his physical and mental infirmities. Other children are so unkind to such a child. All parents, grandparents, and caretakers of children must realize that feeding children such a terrible diet is not being good to them. It's not just having fun or a deed of love, when such heedless permissiveness ruins the health and welfare of another human being. It is destructive behavior on the part of the adult.

Healthy food can be tasty and a delight to enjoy. The richest natural source of chromium is red sour grape powder. It's available as a nutritional supplement, both in powder form and in capsules. It provides 35 percent of the adult requirement for the RDA per teaspoon. For children one or two teaspoons daily can be mixed in soup, yogurt, smoothies, and meat dishes. It can also be added to sandwiches, sprinkled over cereals, or mixed in any drink or even in water. It is totally natural from sun-dried whole sour grapes, so it is virtually impossible to overdose. Food sources are better than the GTF and picolinate chromium or other synthetic formulas. However, even these can be useful when deficiency is pronounced. When deficiency is severe, supplementation may be used for a period of time until blood and tissue levels are stabilized. The food source is most desirable and safe to use every day. Other natural sources of this mineral include the bran/germ of grains, organic liver, and organic eggs.

Zinc

Zinc is an easy mineral to check for deficiency. If the nails have white spots, this is the tell-a-tale sign.

Zinc has many important functions. As is chromium, it is a component of insulin and plays an important role in the function of other hormones as well. It also helps in the removal of CO_2 from the cells. Protein in the skin and collagen require zinc for their synthesis and cellular production. Thus, for normal wound healing adequate levels of zinc are required. Phosphorus could not be readily digested and metabolized without the aid of zinc. Yet, one of the most important functions of this mineral is for the sexual development of the male child and, ultimately, the production of male reproductive fluid.

Severe deficiency can impair male genital development. In girls insufficient zinc may cause the menses to be delayed. If a child loses his/her appetite, taste, or smell, it is normally due to low zinc levels in the cells. When a child gains weight quickly, zinc deficiency will cause stretch marks, especially on the hips and thighs. Also, a noticeable body odor may be present. As mentioned previously, this is easily solved by supplying a liquid calcium, magnesium, and zinc supplement.

Zinc is commonly found in organic meat—especially liver, and in wheat germ, sesame seeds/tahini, peanut butter and peanuts, oregano and thyme, and whole grains. However, regarding the latter, phytates impede its digestion. This is why grains usually act as a zinc antagonist. Thus, the massive intake of whole grains can lead to zinc deficiency. Many plant sources are minimal with pumpkinseeds, alfalfa sprouts, and asparagus supplying the most.

The amount of zinc for infants on a daily basis is around 3 to 5 mg. For children 10 to 15 mg is usually appropriate with teens requiring at least 15 mg daily. The actions of zinc are more effective when it is taken with vitamins A, B_6, and E. Other minerals that facilitate its usage are calcium, copper, cobalt, and phosphorus.

Short stature in children is a significant sign of zinc deficiency. This mineral is also necessary for thyroid hormone production. The connection here is obvious. Zinc is needed for thyroid hormone synthesis, and this hormone controls growth. Likewise, this mineral is needed to activate thyroid hormone.

Along with vitamin A zinc is necessary for protein metabolism. The cells of the body are made up of protein, and that is why growth is affected if these deficiencies are present. Adding zinc-rich foods to the diet and possibly supplements would be beneficial.

Perhaps the best zinc supplement is formulated in Germany. Known as Unizinc, the absorption is superior to others, since it is a chelated zinc aspartate form. Otherwise, keep lots of organic pumpkin seeds around for snacking, and mix them with other organic nuts and seeds such as walnuts, sunflower seeds, hazelnuts, pecans, and peanuts, if tolerated. This nut and seed mixture supplies the zinc and vitamin A, B_6 and vitamin E so the zinc is readily absorbed and effectively used in the body. The nut mixture with toasted sesame seeds added, plus crude sesame oil, which is also rich in vitamin E, can be processed in a blender for a nutritious spread. Add a couple of tablespoons of the crude/remote source sesame oil to the nut/seed mixture, then blend. Add more oil if the nut/seed mixture is too thick to use as a dip or spread. To leave it a bit chunky, just use less oil and less blending time. This mixture and remote source Monukka raisins are delightful on salads, or it is delicious on avocados, celery sticks or apples chunks.

For best results soak the fresh nuts and seeds by covering them with pure water for several hours or even overnight. This causes them to go into sprout mode, and they are easier to digest and utilize in the body. Even toddlers can eat the smooth nut butter, and it is so nutritious and delicious. If the child/children have adrenal symptoms, use sea salt on the nut mix and in the nut/seed butter mixture to taste.

Note: Sun-dried Monukka raisins are one of the richest sources of minerals and other nutrients. At a minimum they supply potassium, sulfur, calcium, iron, and vitamins A, B complex and C. They do contain seeds, which older children can chew and swallow, since they are part of the nourishment package. For young children it is advisable to de-seed them before they eat the raisins. These raisins are huge, so it only takes a few to provide great nourishment and a delicious surprise for the family.

Copper

Copper assists with iron absorption. Both of these minerals are necessary for the formation of red blood cells and hemoglobin. Copper is found throughout the entire body and works with many enzymes in either the buildup or breakdown of tissues. It is mainly concentrated in the brain and vital organs. However, it is found in much higher levels in people with red hair. People with red hair react differently to drugs and anesthesia, and even their blood composition is somewhat different. Likewise, copper works with tyrosine, an amino acid, to form dark skin and hair pigment. It is also a critical nutrient for the repair of elastic tissue, such as the tissue lining the walls of the arteries.

There are many other processes that require copper. Since it is needed for protein metabolism, it is a necessary component for wound healing as well. Bone formation and maintenance is another critical aspect of copper. RNA could not be produced without an adequate level of this mineral. Since copper is needed in the synthesis of phospholipids (fat-related substances like lecithin), it is important for the brain and the myelin sheaths that surround the nerves. The muscles require the breakdown product of vitamin C to form elastin. Without copper this protein could not be formed.

Sources of copper are fairly easy to find. Organic liver is rich in this mineral, and so are soybeans. Unless soy is certified organic, it should not be used. Soy is one of the most highly GMO-contaminated products. Other plant sources of copper include green leafy vegetables, beans, and almonds. Seafood is a good source, but there is also the contamination issue. Infants need around .5 to 1 mg daily and children from 1 to 3 mg.

Too much copper can be toxic. Some of the results of a toxic overload include autism, hyperactivity, depression, mental illnesses, stuttering, insomnia, and hypoglycemia. If too much copper is present in the body, around 10 to 20 mg of zinc or manganese will assist in its elimination through the urine. Molybdenum actually blocks copper absorption.

Usually, copper deficiencies are rare except when children eat only processed and fast foods. Copper and iron deficiency are linked in cases of anemia in children as well as edema and severe protein deficiency. For children with skin sores and wounds that do not heal, copper may be deficient. Breathing problems and generalized weakness may also be signs of insufficiency.

Selenium

Selenium, along with vitamin E, is an important antioxidant. Lipid membranes protect tissues, such as the nerves, heart, and digestive organs, from damage. Selenium protects these lipid membranes from oxidative damage. The elasticity of tissues is preserved by delaying the oxidation of polyunsaturated fatty acids. Here, selenium is crucial. It is also associated with cancer prevention. Glutathione peroxidase, a selenium dependent enzyme, along with vitamin E, protect against a condition in infants where the red blood cells are short-lived. These substances also may prolong the life of white blood cells and increase their protective power.

There is a disease primarily in China called Keshan disease. It is a form of heart disease, and it mostly affects children and women of childbearing age. The main symptom is cardiomyopathy. Muscle pain and tenderness are generally present. With American children eating such poor quality, sugar-laden, refined, GMO-tainted and chemical-infested foods, it is no surprise that so many children and young adults are dying of sudden heart failure.

Selenium insures an adequate oxygen supply, and this is beneficial for the heart. It is also protective for maintaining normal blood pressure and helps to keep arteries clear. It binds with toxic metals and seems to protect the body from assimilating these poisons. It seems to help strengthen the antibodies that neutralize toxins. Selenium is the one mineral that has been found to be protective against cancer. This may be due to the fact that cancer cannot grow in an aerobic environment, and selenium supports oxygen in the cells.

Crib deaths have long been a mystery. Studies are showing that selenium deficiency may be one of the factors responsible for this terrible event. This is because selenium is needed so that the body can properly utilize oxygen.

When severe protein deficiency, medically known as kwashiorkor, is a problem for children, natural protein foods combined with selenium cause a beneficial response quickly. That is why all the money collected to feed those pitiful children with the swollen bellies is not helping them. The white pasty gruel substance that they are given does not have enough protein or selenium to stop the damage of kwashiorkor. It will stop their crying and the hunger pangs but provides little nourishment other than calories. Likewise, vegan children frequently suffer from failure to thrive due to protein, vitamin, and mineral deficiencies. Such deficiencies can be immediately recognized by the coarse, dry texture and lack of sheen of the hair and also poor skin tone.

Toxicity can occur from plant sources and water supplies if too much selenium is in the soil, or it even may be inhaled in polluted industrial areas. Symptoms would include dermatitis, loss of hair, teeth, and nails, fatigue and lethargy, and even paralysis in some cases. If a toxic overdose occurs from a supplement, such as sodium selenite, there may be a high fever, rapid respiration, liver and gastrointestinal disturbances, damage to nerve sheaths, garlic smelling breath and sweat, and even death. Dimethyl selenium, organic selenium, and selenium yeast are the safest forms of supplements.

It is difficult to recommend natural sources, because if there is little to no selenium in the soil, the food will have little to none. There are large areas in the United States that are deficient, and yet parts of Wyoming and the Dakotas have an overabundance of natural selenium. Processing and cooking also deplete minerals from food. However, Brazil nuts are consistently an excellent source of selenium and other foods which may be good sources are brewer's yeast, meats, fish, some grain/cereals, and butter. The average American is either deficient or barely within the normal range of the daily selenium recommendation. Good dietary sources of selenium should be consumed daily with a natural vitamin E source.

Manganese

Manganese is a vital part of the enzyme systems and a catalyst in cell metabolism. It also works with the B complex vitamins to help fight fatigue and apathy. Combined with phosphatase, it is necessary to build strong bones. While it is needed for turning glucose into energy, it is also involved with the formation of fatty acids and fat production. Also, the synthesis of cholesterol is manganese dependent. Cholesterol is needed for a healthy nervous system. It is also required for the proper function of muscles, the brain, and the thyroid gland. Since it is involved in so many enzyme activities, it is expected that manganese is needed for digestion and utilization of nutrients for the entire body. In nursing mothers it improves milk flow.

Manganese deficiency is not overly common, but the joints will make a clicking, popping sound when there is too much or too little in the body. For example, in certain parts of Canada there is so much manganese in the water that the fingernails turn black around the cuticles, and it discolors the cracks and lines of the fingers. It will wash off after a time while cleansing the hands with uncontaminated water. It does take a few weeks for the joints to release the excess manganese.

While there is no required amount, the food content does depend on the degree of availability in the soil and how processed the food is. It is commonly found in fresh unprocessed foods such as green leafy vegetables, peas, beets, nuts and whole grains. A bowl of steamed brown rice with sunflower seeds, raspberries and blackberries, raw honey, and milk is a tasty way to have a delicious warm breakfast full of nourishment and manganese. Also, pulverized hibiscus flower tea is a top source of this mineral.

Fluorine

Fluorine is the most reactive of all elements. As fluoride it is a contaminant added to water supplies. This poison can actually cause the teeth to turn brown and crumble due to toxic overload. It can also cause crumbling of the bones and is, thus, a cause of brittle bones. When in a natural state, as calcium fluoride, it may be safe and even beneficial when combined with calcium and other minerals for the bones and teeth. However, in the water supplies it is added as sodium or aluminum fluoride. This poison accumulates, because it is added repeatedly as the water is recycled. Fluoride is also a common ingredient in most toothpastes and commercial mouthwashes. For small children just learning dental hygiene, they may swallow the toothpaste rather than spitting it out. There are warnings on boxes and tubes not to do so. Therefore, it should be no surprise that there have been deaths recorded for children due to fluoride toxicity. In addition, many dentists apply fluoride treatments.

No other mineral is forced upon the public in this way. A commercial baby food was pulled off the market, because it contained 64 ppm (parts per million) in every jar. The food was cooked in fluoride-contaminated water. Food or beverages should never contain more than .6 ppm to be considered safe for infants and children. Children have developed mottled teeth with as little as .7 ppm, which means they have been poisoned. 64 ppm is a lethal dose.

Fluoride compromises the absorption of calcium, especially in the bones. Yet, calcium is the antidote of choice for fluoride poisoning. So, it is recommend that people who are forced to drink and bathe in this toxic water should use calcium-rich foods and supplements. Even reverse osmosis and steam distillation have not adequately removed such a small molecule. It seems new equipment for removing fluoride has recently been developed. For information call Lifesource Water at 1-800-992-3997.

Molybdenum

Molybdenum is found just about everywhere. In the body it is essential for two enzymes called xanthine oxidase and aldehyde oxidase. Xanthine oxidase helps to move iron from the liver stores, when it is needed elsewhere in the body. Aldehyde oxidase oxidizes fats. This means that when fat is oxidized it is used for a fuel source in the body. The heart is the main organ that uses fat for fuel. Copper metabolism also requires molybdenum. It is generally found in meats, dark green leafy vegetables, unmilled cereal grains, and legumes, but again it depends on soil quality as well as the degree to which the food is processed.

Minerals for health

There are many other minerals which are required in minute amounts. These are known as trace minerals. They are needed for the skin, hair, teeth, and bones. They are also needed for the blood, organs, and all other bodily fluids and tissues. If children are getting a sufficient amount of the major minerals, it is likely that they are also getting a sufficient amount of the trace minerals. To get plenty of these minerals the key is to consume a wide variety of healthy, organic foods and drinks. This must become a standard habit. Junk foods must be avoided, because they contribute nothing to health and a continued state of wellness.

When minerals are in short supply because of poor food quality, a high stress lifestyle, and poor food choices, chronic illness and fatigue (total burn out) or hyperactivity (stuck in overdrive) are certain to occur. The thousands of actions and reactions take place on a minute-by-minute basis in the body. The trillions of cells are unable to thrive and function without the appropriate minerals to make it all happen.

Minerals are the most important components of all the nutrients regarding overall health. These nutrients are also significant for a healthy morale and happiness. Dr. Weston Price traveled to the most remote locations on the earth and studied many cultures. He verified this most significant fact. If the people had an ideal intake of minerals and even if the rest of their overall food intake was limited, still, they remained strong, healthy, happy, and content. Contrast this to Americans who eat large quantities of food and still fail to get the required amounts of nutrients. When refined and processed foods were introduced to these remote villages and deficient foods became a staple part of the diets, all of the diseases of civilization, such as tooth decay, heart disease, diabetes, cancer, tuberculosis, obesity, and arthritis, became the common afflictions of the populations.

Mineral deficiency affects the appearance. It also affects mental powers. Minerals are necessary for the stamina to do physical work and to maintain athletic prowess. Without all their benefits an individual is tired, weak, and apathetic. It has been said that beauty is only skin deep, but nutritionally speaking it also goes all the way to the bone. In fact, bone, spine, and teeth distortions affect the way a person looks. This is certainly related to mineral deficit. How a person functions and how he/she feels on a day-to-day basis is also related. Without the minerals brain function is adversely affected. Thought transmissions are impeded and so are the powers of memory. In trace mineral and major mineral deficiency there is decreased intelligence and mental alertness. Overall, a person is less vibrant. In the mineral deprived the spark of life and vitality are lost. Joy is never at optimal levels. In other words, people are moody and/or morose. Most people function at a level lower than their actual capacity. Today, this is true all over the world.

No doubt, everyone wants the best possible life experiences and health for any child or children under their care. If that is not a priority, people should wait to have a family until this is resolved. This resolution may possibly be achieved with counseling and personal development efforts. For people who are already taking care of children, it is critical to be sure that the entire family is getting the nutrients needed, especially the minerals. Undoubtedly, this will change lives for the better.

I tried an experiment to see how enriching soil with mineral-rich humates from New Mexico would affect food grown in my garden. The garden is located in a somewhat shady area. In the past the tomatoes were always slow to develop and ripen. This last growing season was even cooler than normal and rainy. Though not ideal weather for tomatoes, they grew to be much larger than usual in the humate-enriched soil. Also, they ripened weeks earlier than ever before. However, the best surprise was the fantastic, luscious flavor. They tasted like tomatoes my grandfather grew on mineral-rich soil in the hot sunshine. During this past growing season the main complaint was that it was too cold and wet for the tomatoes to develop their best flavor. Certainly, this was my proof that minerals are mandatory for plants to thrive and even excel under adverse conditions.

The Hunzans in their remote mountain villages are living proof that minerals alone play an important role in creating a super race of people. Their food sources are limited, but their water comes from a mineral-rich ancient glacier. The water is so high in minerals that it has a milky appearance. For years it was a mystery why these people were so physically superior as well as happy and peaceful. The only logical conclusion was first of all densely mineral-rich water. Other important factors were absolutely no processed nutrient-depleted food, and a simple lifestyle in a nurturing community. Going back to these important basics can change life for the better.

Chapter Four

What Makes Kids Thrive

Of course, oxygen and water are the first two most important components that keep the body alive. Likewise, food is also required to nourish the body. Good healthy food will provide the fuel to make a body function and grow and to repair all tissue. When we are sick, the right combination of these natural materials are required for healing. The body heals itself. There are no drugs which magically heal. That is why it is so important to give a body the right tools to use for its own specific needs. Wild plants and herbs plus nourishing whole foods provide the basic essential tools for better health and a calm, productive, and happy life.

There are three major components in food, which nourish human tissues every day. They are commonly known as carbohydrates, proteins, and fats, and each of these substances is important for the welfare, strength, and wellness of the body.

Carbohydrates

The first to be discussed is carbohydrates, which supply energy and heat. When broken down, carbohydrates are converted into glycogen. This substance is stored in the liver for future use as a source of glucose for blood sugar regulation. The body needs blood sugar for a continuous supply of energy and for a balanced body temperature. The brain actually uses at least 20 percent of that energy. Thus, when the blood sugar drops, major personality changes occur as well as physical stresses. The temperamental child, the child who cries frequently, the fat child, the so-called lazy child, the skinny and/or hyper child are all very likely to be low in adrenal reserve. All are also experiencing some form of blood sugar abnormality. These children should avoid simple carbohydrates such as refined sugars, cereals, and junk foods. Their diets should include fresh organic vegetables such as parsley, spinach, collards, kale, turnips and turnip greens, broccoli, green onions, sweet peppers, Brussels sprouts, cauliflower, kohlrabi, endive, cabbage, Chinese cabbage, chives, watercress, dandelions, fennel, garlic, asparagus, radishes, tomatoes, celery and celeriac, romaine lettuce, okra, cucumbers, eggplant, summer squash, artichokes, Jerusalem artichokes, and green beans, since these are low in starch and sugar. However, sea salt must also be liberally allowed to balance out the potassium in these vegetables. Additionally, fresh fruits which are relatively low in sugar, such as kiwi, strawberries and most other berries, grapefruit, melons, unsweetened shredded coconut, avocados, pomegranates, lemons, limes, and papayas, are rich in nutrients and not so destructive to the pancreas and blood sugar mechanisms.

Constant use of simple carbohydrate foods high in sugar negatively affects blood sugar. A diet filled with various types of sugars cause children to have blood sugar swings. This is particularly true of heavily refined products, which are devoid of heath-giving nutrients. Sugar, as in fruit, may be a natural component in the food, or it can be added. Many people are not even aware of the vast amount of sugars of some kind that are added to processed foods and beverages. With high or low blood sugar levels negative reactions are inevitable. These blood sugar extremes cause emotional crises such as crying, uncontrolled behavior, argumentative moods, and angry outbursts. Also, physical impairments occur, such as inability to concentrate, headaches, and nervous stomach, which impede a child's natural quest for learning and achieving. Listlessness, light-headedness, or even fainting spells are blatant signs that blood sugar levels are out of control. These are all danger signs that the glands and organs are being stressed and damaged. Serious health problems will ultimately result from heedless eating and drinking of substandard food and drink.

Simple sugar is digested much faster than most starchy compounds. Starches are known as complex carbohydrates. These complex carbohydrates digest more slowly. Yet, for the sugar sensitive child, starchy foods, especially highly refined ones, are still damaging. When carbohydrates are not completely burned as fuel, the remainder is converted into fat and stored in the body. Americans consume huge amounts of sugar and starch. The results of this dietary dilemma are diseases such as diabetes, heart disease, obesity, and all the other disastrous health consequences that accompany this dietary nightmare. Children have a higher incidence of obesity, diabetes, heart disease, mental and emotional disturbances, asthma, allergy, cancer, and general malnutrition than ever before.

There is another form of beneficial carbohydrate, which is actually indigestible. These substances are called cellulose, gums, hemicelluloses, pectins, and pentosans. They act as sources of fiber in the human body. Fiber is necessary to absorb water. When combined with the other materials in the intestines, it helps to form a softer stool. Plus, the peristaltic action or contractions in the bowel are increased. This stops constipation. Constipation is a common problem for many children today.

Most people are familiar with pectin. Pectin is commonly added to food. It works as a gelling agent. One of its benefits is the reduction and maintenance of cholesterol in the body. This and other types of fiber are filling, and they help quench the appetite. Thus, it is helpful for weight control.

Since both sugar and starch act as sources of energy for the body, they are burned first for fuel. This means they are natural protein sparers. Carbohydrates also cause fats to be fully metabolized. Without the carbs, fat metabolism is incomplete. This causes a reaction known as ketosis. Ultimately, a dangerous condition called acidosis occurs.

A diet rich in carbohydrates requires B vitamins. These vitamins act as coenzymes with the enzymes, which are required for carbohydrate metabolism. When highly processed carbohydrate foods devoid of these required vitamin cofactors are the major calories ingested, the tissues become even more depleted. Thus, the body fails to thrive and function appropriately. This is even more pronounced in growing children and teens. If blood test results indicate high fasting serum triglycerides, it means there has been a prolonged excessive intake of carbohydrates, especially from sucrose (table sugar).

When considering what to eat and why, there is a new book called *The Body Shape Diet,* by Dr. Cass Ingram. Hormones play a huge role in what an individual can and cannot digest and utilize. Certain hormone types are less tolerant of sugar and other refined carbohydrates. Children are born with these signs and features associated with the hormone types. The book is amazingly accurate. This analysis is a great help to determine the endocrine needs of children and adults. So many difficulties can be eliminated with this knowledge. This book is a must have.

Still, scientific degrees and massive research are not required to understand that a chronic excess of lifeless, chemical infested, refined junk will not benefit any body. Growing children will not thrive on such garbage. In this developmental stage their needs are even more significant than adult requirements.

Obese individuals often use excess food for emotional reasons as well for nourishment. However, so much which passes for food in the American culture provides virtually nothing beneficial for the physical body. It is just filler. Thus, for many, who are in various stages of overweight, their bodies are driven to eat to try to fulfill physiological needs. These people cannot easily stop eating, because their physical requirements are not being met by the foods they are eating. Quality, not quantity, should be the focus on food for everyone. High quality organic food must be used as nourishment for the organs and tissues. The endless junk, which has been used as a pacifier for hurts and emotional pain, contributes nothing worthwhile. Refined carbohydrates, such as chocolate, cakes, pies, candies, chips, crackers, cookies, and the like, are the usual tasty offenders in this case. Parents, *please* do not use treats and goodies as motivators and rewards for desired behavior. Adults with food hang-ups should never inflict them on youngsters. A strong and healthy body is one of the finest treasures a person can enjoy. Life is so much easier and productive for an emotionally and physically strong individual. To develop this strength, the right diet for a person's hormone type is a must. The best food possible should be consumed. For those who think they cannot afford healthy food, remember this: it is better to eat small amounts of excellent food than huge amounts of poor food. Actually, the body does not require much food to survive, especially when it is high quality, nourishing, and based on the individual's exact physical requirements. (See Dr. Ingram's *The Body Shape Diet.*)

Protein

For children to properly grow and develop, a diet rich in protein is mandatory. Dr. Martin Eastwood from the University of Edinburgh maintains that protein from animal sources is digested and absorbed more easily and completely than vegetable sources. He further states that animal proteins supply more amino acids and small peptides than do vegetable proteins. Of all the types of animal protein range fed buffalo is probably the safest natural source, with organic lamb being next. Other protein sources from organic/range fed beef, organic poultry, such as chicken, turkey, and duck, as well as wild game may be acceptable. However, with wild creatures there is a concern, since they are now eating GMO-contaminated grains and other forage. These wild animals are developing terrible wasting diseases which are killing them. Today, it is very difficult to know what is safe to eat.

Eggs and dairy products also provide all the essential amino acids, but no doubt, they must be from organic sources. The digestion and absorption efficiency of egg protein is approximately 85 to 90 percent, which is excellent. However, casein in dairy products and gluten in grains are resistant to the action of pancreatic enzymes, and digestion is impeded. Raw royal jelly on a daily basis as a complete protein source is an option. It provides all of the essential amino acids, which build and repair cells. It is easy to digest and assimilate especially for the young and the elderly. Unfortunately, an adequate amount of high quality royal jelly as a major protein source is rather expensive. Raw royal jelly is difficult to use when traveling, because it requires special handling. Fortunately, there is a naturally stabilized raw form. It looks like chocolate pudding. Yet, it requires no refrigeration. Therefore, it is easy to transport, since it does not spoil like the kind that requires refrigeration. This stabilized form is also much more palatable than the frozen raw royal jelly. Most children readily consume it without a fuss, and it is especially desirable for children who need extra nourishment. This form of royal jelly readily mixes in smoothies, yogurt, cooked cereals, and pudding.

How the body uses protein

Since protein is such an important part of the diet, it is helpful to somewhat understand how it works in the body. Protein is made up of amino acids. Amino acids are the building blocks of the human body. Of the 22 amino acids at least eight of them are essential. The word essential says it all. These particular amino acids must be supplied almost every day to survive and be healthy. Some of them can be synthesized in the body, but if any are missing, this process is halted. Plants usually provide an incomplete supply of amino acids, especially lysine, methionine, cystine, tryptophan, and threonine. Protein from animal sources provides all the necessary amino acids. There is no question that it is complete. However, overcooking can adversely alter protein structure. All of the amino acids are mandatory for growing, developing children.

Every cell requires protein, and how the amino acids are combined determines the type of protein. There are many uses in the body for these important components. The following is a partial list of how protein broken down into amino acids is utilized in the body:

- amino acids make durable and malleable skin
- ligaments, tendons, and muscles are formed from amino acids
- the lens of the eye, the vitreous fluid inside the eye, and the retina are made of a combination of amino acids
- capillaries, veins, and arteries are made from amino acids
- amino acids combine to make up the entire nervous system
- cholesterol and amino acids form brain cells
- the bones require collagen made from amino acids for their structure
- the cells which make up the immune system, including the natural killer cells, are formed from amino acids
- fingernails, toenails, and hair are made from amino acids
- joint material is derived from amino acids
- hormones, enzymes, antibodies, and vitamins are produced from amino acid
- bodily fluids are made up of various amino acids
- amino acids combine to heal cuts and wounds
- amino acids are needed in the formation of DNA
- amino acids help regulate water in the body and the acid/base balance

Infants and children need to replenish their amino acid supply every day. During infancy the protein content of the body is around 11% and increases to around 15%. By age four the body protein stabilizes at around 18% to 19% and remains at that level throughout adulthood. Mother's milk provides the perfect protein content for the infant, especially when the mother is well nourished. When other foods are given to the infant, the amount of protein must be increased to adjust for the decrease of milk consumed. Children will increasingly need from around 23 grams of protein to as high as 46 grams as teenagers. All eight essential amino acids must be consumed.

If children and teens are very active or have high stress lives, they lose nitrogen in their urine and require more protein. Other factors which affect nitrogen balance include fever, infections, and injuries. Slow healing wounds, failure to grow, frequent infections, brittle nails, and poor hair are symptoms of amino acid deficiencies.

Normally, proteins must be broken down into amino acids for the body to be able to use them appropriately. Newborn babies are the exception. They actually absorb whole proteins. Thus, proteolytic enzymes develop rapidly, which are the backbone of immunological development in the infant. This is why mother's milk is the most perfect food for an infant, since this compatible source of maternal nutrients facilitates rather than challenges the infant's developing system. It is important to note that using synthesized formulas and feeding solid foods/cereals too early can cause immune dysfunction and allergy reactions. This is likely due to the infant's ability to absorb whole proteins, including those which are not compatible. Cow's milk is especially troublesome.

Fat

People have been programmed to believe that all fat is bad. Yet, the body requires fat for energy. Fats and lipids liberate a greater amount of heat than carbohydrates and proteins. This concentrated energy source contains more carbon and hydrogen and less oxygen than carbohydrates and proteins. All cells except the red blood cells and the cells of the central nervous system can readily use the fatty acids for fuel.

Low-fat diets and fat-free diets are dangerous. If a nursing mother eats only low-fat foods or little to no fat, the baby will fail to grow and may even lose weight. Severe eczema is also usually present. Infants with very resistant eczema usually respond immediately to linoleic acid added to their diets.

Essential fatty acids must be in the diet of every living being. The body is unable to synthesize the essential fatty acid known as linoleic acid. However, it is commonly found in both plant and animal sources. Linolenic and arachidonic acids are also needed for the body to function and thrive. Other essential fatty acid deficiency symptoms are dermatitis, increased metabolic rate, craving for water and water-retention, plus drying and flaking of the skin. Many bottle fed babies exhibit essential fatty acid deficiencies, as well as infants and children fed fat-free intravenous fluids in hospitals.

The fatty acids have numerous activities. The fatty acids in phospholipids help maintain the integrity of all the cells. They help to make the skin soft and supple. They are also needed in the use, transport, and excretion of cholesterol. Prostaglandins are important in pain, infection, and inflammation response, and fatty acids are also a component in their formation.

The body uses fat for padding. It acts as a shock absorber. Since it is an insulator, it helps the body to maintain the proper temperature. Fat actually keeps the organs in position within the body. Too much fat is not good for the health. Yet, too little fat is also a danger, since fat is the fuel required for the heart.

Fat makes food taste and smell good. It gives a nice, creamy texture to food. Importantly, fat creates a feeling of being satisfied. Children with weight problems should not be denied healthy fatty foods such as avocado, cold-pressed oils such as pumpkinseed oil, sesame seed oil, and extra virgin olive oil. Walnuts, sunflower seeds, Brazil nuts, and almonds are frequently avoided because of the calories. Yet, they provide a wealth of nourishment.

Needless to say, fast food junk foods and deep-fried foods contain the damaging kinds of fat that harm the arteries, skin, and heart. Without the good natural fats in the diet the fat soluble vitamins A, D, E, and K could not be absorbed and used in the body. This huge consumption of fast foods accounts for many vitamin deficiencies today.

There is a great variation of the amount of fat consumed throughout the world. Today, in the United States around 45% of the total calories ingested are from some form of fat. Actually, around 33% or about one third of the calories as healthy fat in the daily diet is better utilized and tolerated. Obesity is at an all-time high among men, women, and children. Poor eating habits are the cause.

Children acquire their eating habits from their families and their surroundings. This includes other kids, school, meals eaten out, home-delivered pizza, etc. So much of the so-called food today is synthetic. At many events and places of entertainment cheese is not cheese. It is made from a chemical slurry plus refined oils. No one even wants to know what the hot dogs or other mystery meats contain. French fries contain many ingredients other than potatoes, including propylene glycol. This is also known as antifreeze. It gives them a crunchy texture. Yes, those ice cream bars are mostly frozen chemicals too. Yet, this is what the kids eat and then beg for more. This is because it is what they know, a taste they understand. Furthermore, it is accepted by their peers.

Fresh, raw, organic or wild foods are the only worthwhile consumables that will serve their bodies well. Make it "uncool" to eat the dangerous garbage designed to attract their attention. It certainly does nothing to nourish their bodies. If they are strong and healthy due to eating good food, they will not crave the junk. That is why it is important to start good eating habits during infancy.

Carbohydrates, proteins, and fats are all-important substances for growth, development, and energy. There are always great debates among the nutrition experts about the percentages of each of these three food components that are required in the daily diet. For children a wide variety of wholesome, organic natural foods is most important. With small helpings of a variety of foods children are likely to develop a taste for a wider selection of foods as adults. They also gain a wider range of important nutrients. The craving for synthetic foods and those which are called partitioned foods is virtually nonexistent, when they are not consumed on a daily basis. Partitioned foods include any food which has been refined. Some of these familiar foods include white rice, white flour, skim milk, and white sugar. Frequently, this processing is done to increase the shelf life and profitability factor. It is more profitable because the bran, fats, and such, which are derived from processing food, are sold as separate products. Whipped toppings, fake cheeses, coffee creamer, and margarine are examples of synthetic foods. Major alterations (partitioning) of a natural substance reduce or eliminate nutritional value. Sugar and junk food, if ever used, should be allowed only on rare occasions. This is not being mean. It is being protective and responsible, so that children are healthy and grow to their fullest potential. Children must learn that fake foods are harmful.

As we co-op with the farmers, the prices are more than reasonable for organic food. The farmers are also assured that what they grow will be sold. Therefore, it is cheaper than going to grocery stores and far better and fresher. It was once a rare treat to find an organic farmer to buy food from, but it is becoming increasingly common. It is in our best interests to buy as much food this way as possible.

Some farmers cannot afford to pay the fees for organic certification. Yet, many follow organic farming practices by using no pesticides, herbicides, or chemical fertilizers. Plus, if they use heirloom, non-GMO seeds, then it is safe to buy their products. Visit the farm to observe their practices.

Also growing food is such a fantastic experience for the entire family. It is very reasonable if the seeds are collected from organic foods and allowed to air dry. Then, the seeds are sprouted indoors early in the spring. It is safe to plant them outside after the last frost. Most people are not on farms, but chickens are allowed as pets in some towns. This is a great way to have fresh eggs every day. However, this really does depend on the location and how friendly the neighbors are. Recently, in a township near Chicago the people in charge refused to let a family have a tiny goat. She was providing milk for the family. It seems she had much better manners than the local dogs, and no one had complained about them. The family and their friends were highly attached to her. All were saddened to lose such a lovely companion and her gift of milk. It's shameful, when laws are about control without the benefit of common sense.

More and more chemicals, medicines, synthetic foods, genetically engineered foods and thousands of additives are introduced into children's diets and lives every year. Today, more children have severe health challenges than ever before. Children can still have fine health and superior mental and physical development. However, they must be taught to avoid what is designed to attract their attention but manufactured with no intent to nourish them. This is criminal capitalism, when human welfare is ignored.

The majority of processed food companies are only concerned with making vast sums of money. That is why the Slow Food movement, which began in Italy, is an important organization. The Slow Food groups support small farmers, who grow healthy and beautiful food. These groups further assist the small co-ops, which make superior food products such as extra virgin olive oil and superb olives, fire-roasted artichoke hearts, luscious sun-dried cherry tomatoes in extra virgin olive oil, pesto, spaghetti sauces, whole grain spaghetti, raw whole milk cheeses, and so much more. Then they help the farmers take their products to market. The food is delicious and nutritious. Some fine examples of this extraordinary food are available on the internet. One great brand named Seggiano has many choices. These foods are available at www.Americanwildfoods.com. These products are pure, tasty food full of nutrients instead of chemicals. They are a delight to the palate, body, and soul.

Chapter Five

Children at Risk

Poisoning our world and our children

This is a different world today. The contaminants found in food, water, and air are continually increasing. Meanwhile, a diminishing amount of natural nutrients are contained in the soil. Phyllis Pierpont, an admirable lady and natural farmer on the plus side of 80 years, says that, currently, farmers burn off the stubble and plant material rather than let it degrade to feed the soil. It is easier to pour on the chemicals. For example, the canola farmers spray a deadly pesticide on the crops in the middle of the night to kill army worms. After this nerve poison is sprayed, it is so deadly that animals wandering through the area will be dead before they are half way through the field. All the farmers who use these evil chemicals are sick. These chemicals were originally created as bio-warfare weapons. These poisons do not just disappear. If there is any doubt that you and your children are eating, drinking, and breathing such poisons, then you are deluding yourself.

Children are always vulnerable, but especially so from conception to around five years of age. This is when these deadly chemicals cause growth and developmental disorders. Also, brain lesions and nerve damage cause learning and behavioral disorders and impede mental development. Furthermore, it sets the stage for debilitating diseases such as diabetes and cancer.

According to the Safer Pest Control Project pesticide exposure is common for more than 13 million American children in day care centers. Sixty-three percent of children under five attend day care around 37 hours per week. Nicolle Tulve, lead researcher with the EPA's National Exposure Research Laboratory, found at least one pesticide in every day care center. These can be from bug sprays to lawn chemicals used on landscape and playgrounds. These poisons drift into the buildings and collect on all public areas. Thus, these deadly chemicals contaminate all surfaces, including toys, desks, windows and floors. They are found on children's clothing, their shoes, and even on the children themselves. Most children are exposed on a daily basis. The half-life or length of time these deadly chemicals remain toxic in the environment are for weeks, months, and even years. Now, from the constant bombing in Afghanistan and Iraq, the DU (depleted uranium) is poisoning not only these lands, but also the rest of the world. The half-life of that disastrous substance is beyond count.

Parents must contact the schools and request safer ways of dealing with pests indoors and also outdoor applications. Ask for a materials-data-safety sheet, the date of the last spraying, and a notification when any spraying is to be conducted.

Children exposed to deadly chemicals need help to remove these vile substances from the cells and tissues of their bodies. Wild raw green juices, such as burdock, nettles, dandelion, and chickweed juices, contain nutrients and enzymes to help rid the liver and other tissues of these toxic substances. For small children even a few drops three times daily are beneficial. For older children a teaspoonful two to three times daily may be necessary depending on exposure. Other helpful preventive measures are to make sure children learn to wash their hands frequently and remove their shoes when entering the home. These chemicals are silent killers. They are readily found on our most personal belongings and in our homes and cars. If you or your children have unexplained symptoms, consider the possibility of pesticide poisoning. Some of the most common symptoms include headaches, nausea, anemia, indigestion, loss of appetite, crawling sensation on the skin, nerve damage, sleep disturbances, inability to concentrate, and blistered skin not due to herpes.

It just doesn't make sense that the EPA banned the use of the toxic pesticide lindane for the application on seed crops, yet, it is still commonly used on children to kill head lice and scabies. The FDA allows it to be the major component in *prescription* shampoos and lotions designated for the heads and bodies of these delicate little souls. Remember that chemicals are readily absorbed through the skin. This is particularly true of the scalp, which has a rich blood supply. There are completely natural products which destroy the vermin, and they are totally safe for all ages. Always seek such safe and effective options. Hopefully, such products are available in fine health food stores.

The vaccination myth

Parents are besieged to vaccinate their children from the moment they are born. Many times in hospitals newborns are rushed off and jabbed with hepatitis B shots without the parents' knowledge or consent. One mother always gave birth to her babies at home assisted by a midwife. She chose to do this to protect those babies from unwanted medications and procedures. However, for one pregnancy her midwife was not available. Therefore, she selected a highly recommended hospital for delivery. This experienced mother carefully instructed the doctor and nurses before the birth that no vaccinations or drugs were to be given to the infant. They did it anyhow, and the child has suffered from a chronic skin disease his entire life. All of her other unvaccinated children are strong and healthy.

No research has been done to determine if these vaccinations are safe or even effective. Yet, it is a common practice, and the claims are profuse. The only certain benefit is a monetary one for their makers.

Vaccinations, despite what you may have read or been told, are not the miracle that they have been made out to be. Dr. Cass Ingram explains the danger of damaging the immune system with these foreign and toxic substances. For an exposé on the danger of vaccinations read his book *Natural Cures for Killer Germs*. To learn about the polio vaccination and sugar cube hoax, read Ingram's *The Cause for Cancer Revealed*. Dr. Sherri Tenpenny also continues to write extensively about the dangers of vaccinations. She has evidence-based books, papers, and audio and video materials. Dr. Doris Rapp is a famous pediatrician, allergist, and environmental medical specialist. She is a fine doctor who champions responsible and safe medical care for children. Her books are *Is This Your Child's World? You Can Fix the Schools and Homes That are Making Your Children Sick,* and *Our Toxic World: A Wake Up Call.* The books are packed with information every informed family should know. This valuable information is available on the internet, libraries, bookstores, and health food stores.

While most people believe that vaccinations are mandatory, in actuality, parents can choose not to do so. Most certainly, doctors, nurses, and school officials harass the parents to inoculate their children. In Appendix B of this book there is a document which you can copy, sign, and give to the school for exemption of vaccinations. They won't like it, but they must accept it in most states. Don't be afraid to take a stand.

Children who do get the miserable inoculations will have viral shedding. This shedding exposes others to the viruses. Others can get sick from such exposure. So, on vaccination days at school it is wise to keep children at home. For a day or two afterwards unvaccinated children must avoid contact with these contaminated children.

There is always the argument from the vaccination proponents that unvaccinated children may somehow imperil the vaccinated children. Common sense will destroy that argument. If vaccinated children are supposed to be protected against diseases, how can unvaccinated children be a threat?

All children can keep their immune systems strong with healthy organic food and drinks. Since body composition is mostly water, clean filtered water is a must. Dr. Doris Rapp recently said at a medical conference that clean, pure water can relieve most anything. While traveling, I am always armed with an array of supplements that keep me going. Close to the end of a health conference, I had used or given away to fellow travelers every supplement. Then, I began to feel ill. Remembering what Dr. Rapp said, I began sipping on bottled water all evening and intermittently throughout the night. By morning I was feeling much better. For everyone adequate rest, good hygiene, supplements that support the immune system, clean water, positive thoughts and heartfelt prayers are health building and sustaining necessities.

Poisons in the water

In 1985 I purchased my first water filter for the kitchen sink. For me and many others Mr. Ewald Ereshmann, the inventor of this special unit, created a totally new awareness about the importance of truly clean water. He explained the dangers that lurk in what is thought to be pure. Just because there isn't anything visibly floating in the water, it is believed that it is fit for bathing and consumption. What he proved to me with a pile of documents, testing, and research is that minimal filtration is done—only the big stuff is removed. This means that cities dump raw sewage into the local water sources such as the rivers and lakes. Then, this recycled water is chlorinated and fluoridated, and that is what is coming out of the faucet. There is no quality control for purity. Water is further contaminated with manufacturing waste, nuclear material, fertilizers and other chemicals, pesticide and herbicide runoff, and muck from massive hog farms. Furthermore, hospital waste and blood products are a major danger as is the urine of those who consume multitudes of drugs everyday. The list of nasty, foul material contaminating the public water supplies is endless.

Mr. Ereshmann listed over one hundred toxic substances in the water. He worked with cities and farms to build systems which truly filtered the water with a combination of high grade carbon, magnetic devices, and very fine filters.

He found dead birds and even dead dogs in those big water storage towers that are so commonly seen. They are not pristine and clean as is hoped and believed. That is one reason why high levels of chlorine are used.

A young man contacted me for help. His father while working in the water purification plant in Chicago contracted leukemia. He further confirmed that since no decontamination/filtration is done to the water, chlorine was the chemical of choice to destroy any major pathogens. Chlorine added to the water is terribly toxic, but since it is a gaseous substance it does dissipate to a degree as it is carried through the pipes. However, the closer a home is to the water facility, the higher the level of chlorine is in the water.

Chlorine itself is a dangerous substance. However, it also combines with already toxic chemicals to form substances such as trichloromethane, a deadly compound. This is in all public drinking and bathing water, since it is unfiltered.

If at all possible, do have filtration units for the kitchen sink and the shower/bath. Better yet, a whole house unit provides clean water for the family and clean pipes and fixtures for the entire house. One of the best systems is made by Lifesource Water Systems in Pasadena, California. For more information call 1-800-992-3997. The toxic substances found in water are absorbed through the skin. An adult absorbs up to two pounds of water when bathing. Children are also like little sponges. Always keep in mind that children are more susceptible to the damaging effects of all chemicals and poisons.

Unfortunately, one of the major toxins in the water is added purposely. Every time the water passes through the water treatment plant, fluoride is added to it. That means the parts per million of fluoride just keep steadily increasing. It is also added to every commercial toothpaste and mouthwash. Fluoride is supposed to prevent cavities. Yet, in March of 2006 a panel of dentists, toxicologists, and epidemiologists gathered together by the NRC (National Research Council) concluded that fluoride levels allowed in public drinking water are too high. They also determined that children drinking water containing these high levels of fluoride permitted by the EPA are actually damaging their teeth. It causes the teeth to be splotched and streaked with yellow and brown stains. Frequently, the enamel becomes pitted, and this actually creates cavities. There are other dangers of high fluoride intake such as lowered IQ levels. Furthermore, exposure to high levels of fluoride weakens bones over time. This may ultimately cause an increase in fractures and osteoporosis. Even a rare form of bone cancer may be activated, especially in young boys. Dr. Ionel Rapaport, while at the University of Wisconsin, reported that there is a direct relationship of mongolism and fluoridated drinking water. Dr Hardy Limeback, head of preventive dentistry at the University of Toronto, states in the NRC's fluoride report that "it (fluoride) could turn out to be one of the top 10 mistakes of the 21st century."

Warnings on toothpaste state that if children swallow fluoride to seek medical attention or call the Poison Control Center. If this isn't sufficient proof that it is harmful, then, what could really convince anyone? Fluoride accumulates in body tissues. Do not use dental hygiene products laced with fluoride. Health stores carry products without fluoride. Request fluoride free products, if stores do not have them. Unfortunately, what has already been added will contaminate public water supplies for generations to come.

This is not new information. Many communities have fought against adding this toxin to their water supply for years. Some win, but most of them lose. After all, it is a most effective, efficient, and lucrative way to dispose of the aluminum fluoride, an industrial waste product. This is another example of criminal capitalism. Meanwhile, in many countries across Europe fluoridation is banned.

How to protect your children's teeth from excess fluoride

Most home filtration systems cannot remove fluoride. Bottled mineral water with no additional fluoride may be the answer until proper filtration can be arranged. Even that is no guarantee, since there are no regulations on bottled water. Some common brands have been found to be no more than bottled tap water. If it is labeled spring water bottled at the source, one can hope that it is truly pure water. Check the website www.prevention.com/water for bottled water recommendations. Fluoridation should end now.

Children must consume healthy, mineral-rich food and supplements to nourish the bones and teeth. Organic fruits and vegetables have higher mineral levels and are not sprayed with pesticides which leave high fluoride residues.

The government deems that 1 part per million of fluoride is considered to be safe in drinking water. Yet, the Academy of Pediatrics recommends that fluoride should not be supplemented during the first six months of life. Thus, municipal water and infant water laced with fluoride are dangerous for babies. It is best to make baby food in a blender with organic food or buy organic baby food. Avoid chicken-based baby food. It may contain high levels of fluoride from the bone residue of the chicken during the deboning process. Baby formula, cereals, or food must only be prepared with non-fluoridated water. Never use soda pop and other commercial drinks and juices made with fluoridated water.

Common symptoms of fluoride poisoning are salivation, nausea, vomiting, diarrhea, and abdominal pain. Chronic signs include weakness, shallow respiration, tremors, spasms, and convulsion. Brain, kidney, heart, and circulatory damage, crumbling teeth, bone weakness/cancer, diabetes, human enzyme destruction, and endocrine gland damage also result from fluoride contamination. See www.fluorideaction.net and www.fluoridealert.org. Read the full story in *The Fluoride Deception,* by Christopher Bryson.

Sugar—the real culprit

You constantly are told that salt is the killer. Yet, sodium and chloride are important electrolytes in the body. People would die without them. Never is one word mentioned in the public forum that sugar is a problem. Even the huge nutrition conventions that banned sugar in the past, now often feature the sugar companies as their main speakers. Yes, even they have been bought out.

There is a vast attack on the use of salt, even properly prepared sea salt. However, the salt slayers never voice one word about the dangers of sugar. In fact, sugar is built into the food pyramid as a normal part of the diet. Some even tout it to be better than many natural foods. This is regarding the glycemic index. The glycemic index is a measure of how fast sugar or starch is digested and absorbed by the body. Starch must be broken down into sugar before it can be absorbed. Therefore, the absorption rate of simple sugar is swift compared to a complex starch which causes blood sugar to rise slowly. Frequently, it is denied that sugar causes countless health problems and diseases. Yet, it is far more dangerous and destructive than salt. To prevent children from being nearsighted, nervous, and unable to concentrate and learn, sugar must be avoided. It can cause a child to become obese or too thin depending on the degree of damage to the liver and blood sugar mechanisms. The more that sugar is consumed, the more the liver is damaged. This results in blood sugar disorders and also allows the blood to become overloaded with fungus. Sugar is food for fungus, and fungal infections are common among children. Furthermore, sugar actually causes depletion of vital vitamins and minerals. Eventually, these malnourished youngsters are unable to cope, and they become hyperactive nightmares or limp and lifeless dishrags. Of course, both types are unable to excel to their highest potential. Physically, these small sugar addicts are cursed with a mouthful of cavities. Then these cavities are filled with toxic mercury fillings. No parents could possibly wish to inflict all of this misery on their children. Unfortunately, these are the typical results when children are allowed to consume sugar every day. Oh yes, if they are also deprived of sea salt as well, then this terrible dilemma will be topped off with adrenal exhaustion.

What can be done about it? How discretionary income is spent is a personal choice. Spending decisions determine what kind of health status children will have throughout a lifetime. It is necessary to be educated to make the wisest choices possible. Industry only researches how to make a product most desirable or, preferably, addictive. Then, it must be as cheap as possible. This is all done for the greatest financial return. Not one moment of caring is given to the health and welfare of the family. The only way the family can control what is in the market place is with buying power. Remember, kids need care, and so do you.

In the past diabetes was called sugar diabetes. Now it is known as diabetes mellitus type II (the more common form) and juvenile diabetes is type I. Even in the natural health arena practitioners are diverted from calling sugar the main culprit of the diabetes disaster that afflicts hundreds of thousands of people today. The mainstream practitioners call this huge increase in blood sugar diseases a true mystery. This is beyond nonsense. It is the manufacturers' crime against humanity.

Foods are refined and filled with additives to make them last indefinitely on the shelf. Ironically, the food industry claims that the public demands a consistently uniform appearance. Additionally, processed foods are researched and developed for taste and eye appeal. There is no thought or consideration given to nutrient content or health giving properties. However, there is a way to change this. Consumer demand actually could alter the way food is manufactured for the better. Every time nutritious, wholesome foods free of endless additives are purchased, that counts as a vote for better quality. Always seek truly organically grown or even wild food gathered from nature. Why not have a garden, even just an herb garden in the window? There is nothing better than fresh picked food.

I became the legal guardian for my nephew when he was 14. Being adamantly determined to help him acquire better eating habits, we went to the largest health food store in the Chicago area. He asked for breakfast cereal. I told him he could get whatever he liked as long as it did not contain any form of sugar. His father died of complications from diabetes, his mother has severe blood sugar issues, and he also has that propensity. It seemed like the young fellow was gone forever, so I headed over to the cereal aisle to see what was causing the delay. He claimed that the boxed cereals, except for the kind that required cooking, all contained some sort of sugar. I said something like you've got to be kidding me and began to read the labels on the boxes myself. This was truly an ordeal, because the cereal aisle is about twenty feet long and over six feet high. Between the two of us we read every label. He ended up with puffed rice and was not at all thrilled with that choice. The point is it doesn't matter where you shop, because the food is totally loaded with some form of sugar/sweetener. Even tomato sauce, condiments, vegetables, breads and rolls, yogurt, sausages, herring, fake milks and flavored milks, fake eggs, salt, crackers, bottled teas and other drinks, dried fruit, nuts, chips, and so much more are contaminated with some form of sugar. Many chefs claim that the flavor of most every dish is not as good without sugar. I heartily disagree. The rest of the civilized world does not use the mountains of sugar and sweeteners that are consumed in the United States. Unfortunately, this is changing. They are beginning to catch up with American sugar cravings along with obesity and other related diseases due to constant sugar consumption.

The first book I read about the dangers of sugar was *Sugar Blues,* by William Duffy. It was shocking to read about the processing procedures that manufacturers employ, which leave no nutrients in the white granular addictive substance known as sugar. It not only gives you no nourishment, but it also robs the body of its vital stores of vitamins and minerals. Today, government regulations are more draconian than ever before in the name of so-called consumer welfare. However, it does not apply to the megalithic industries, which have hundreds of lobbyists supporting their causes. The huge industries through their political clout control most government actions. The government regulatory agencies ignore blatant corruption. These agencies make sure that mega-manufacturers have little to no competition from small upstart businesses. This is especially so if those small businesses focus on the true health and welfare of the people. Consumers must support those businesses which are earth friendly and people proactive. This is especially important, since more than 70% of the money everyone works so hard for is collected as some form of taxation. This includes city, county, state and federal taxes, fees, licenses, penalties, and tolls.* Any remaining amount of money that is left should be spent carefully as a meaningful tool to exert a collective power for better health and to support any other needs of humanity and future generations. Everyone must work together now, so that there is a future for people on this planet, a happy and blessed one.

*Note: taxes include all forms of state and federal taxation to include income taxes, all forms of sales taxes, property taxes, "sin" taxes for cigarettes, alcohol and gambling, license fees to include everything from fishing and hunting licenses, driver's license, automobile license, city stickers, business licenses and much more; death taxes: probate, estate, inheritance—soon to rise exponentially by 2010; tolls on roads and bridges, excise taxes (war tax), personal property taxes, wealth taxes—only the billionaires supposedly don't pay taxes—the moderately well-to-do pay up to 50% of their wages on income taxes/alternative taxes alone; transportation taxes, surcharges on fuel, hotel/entertainment taxes, phone bill taxes, capital gains tax, luxury taxes, federal and state public park fees, service taxes, insurance fees and social security taxes, unemployment tax, worker's compensation tax, Medicare tax, school tax, real estate tax, building permit tax, well permit tax, septic permit tax, utility taxes, severance tax, privilege tax, use tax, intangible taxes, inventory tax, recreational vehicle taxes, pet license taxes, road usage taxes, IRS penalties and interests, federal and state government fines and penalties, municipal fines and penalties, gasoline/diesel taxes at the pumps, seat belt fines, license plate fines, parking fines, speeding fines, and there are *many* more taxes, fees, fines, and licenses not listed. If enforced federal health care is made mandatory in the United States, wages will be garnished or there is a threat of prison if one does refuse to join and pay a percentage of personal income. It is not free health care as people are led to believe. So that means there are always more plans afoot to reduce personal wealth and discretionary income.

The endless collection of revenues are certainly an infringement on personal liberties and rights. So much of the money collected is wasted or funneled off to special interest groups and wars. Power and control are the motives for this financial catastrophe.

There is a constant effort to raise tax rates. If money already collected was correctly used, it would be needless to inflict these endless raises on the populace. The people who are supposed to be our leaders are out of control. Future generations are burdened with debts in the trillions of dollars as money is handed out to a favored few. Still, millions are out of work and losing their homes. Yet, all of this can be changed by everyone intensely focusing on the ideal life for the family. Remember to do the vision board and apply explicit pictures (snap shots, pictures from magazines, brochures, etc.) of all that is desired. This could be a picture of the perfect home and ideal means of transportation, the best schools for the children, money and investments, something indicating an ideal career, and, most importantly, any and all spiritual advancements. What is most desirable is anything that is for the greatest good of all people on this planet. That means willing cooperation by all, not universal mandates by a few. When personal desires coincide with that, everyone benefits. When everyone focuses on the highest good for all, then we will have reached a higher spiritual level. Only then can the planet change for the better. Remember that change for the better starts with one person at a time. Be that one person, be that change for the better, and help others to join the quest for the best.

Sugar will not make a child grow. It will not make him/her happy, at least for very long. It may raise the blood sugar for a sugar high, but then it will drop like a rock. Then all the consequences begin such as nausea, shakiness, headache, dry mouth, feeling faint or actually fainting, irritability, cloudy thinking, inability to remember, fatigue or hyperactivity depending on the person, blurred or impaired vision, crying spells, temper tantrums, inability to concentrate, and so much more. It does not increase intelligence, because it robs the body of those important B vitamins. Depression and behavioral problems are directly related to this most common chemical. Yet, rather than remove sugar from the diet, parents are told to give a "troublesome" child more chemicals/mind-altering drugs. Once this routine is started, the child has little chance of getting off the drug merry-go-round, legal or illegal. Find other options. Do not give up. If help or guidance is needed, seek it. There are holistic practitioners who can help people out of the common public rut. Spiritual guidance is also an absolute necessity. It is written in the Bible, "Seek and ye shall find,"—the help that is needed. No matter what one's belief system includes, these words apply to all souls.

Poisoned, processed foods

In 2008 tons of peanut butter were recalled, because it contained the bacteria salmonella. A company in Georgia supplied the majority of the peanut butter for all types of packaged snack foods. Some 500 people were sickened, and eight deaths occurred. Likewise, tons of ground beef have been contaminated with E. coli and other bacteria. The recalls have been so massive, that companies have gone out of business. Undoubtedly, cleanliness is a factor. However, the poor quality of the food products due to factory farming methods are also a factor. Factory farming means that deadly pesticides, herbicides, chemicals, and GMO-tainted seeds are the accepted formula for food production. That is why the resulting foods are so easily contaminated.

Furthermore, is this just another way to push the agenda for irradiating all processed food? It has been proven that irradiation destroys nutrients, such as vitamin C and E, as well as the carotenes. Plus, does it really kill bad bacteria and fungus? According to a number of investigators this process fails to truly sterilize germs and, instead, creates mutant ones. This was clearly demonstrated by the University of Iowa researchers, whereby *Candida albicans* was subjected to irradiation. Here, the candida, which normally exists in two forms, was converted into 90 different mutants. Other studies show that while the irradiation causes the bacteria to burst and splatter, it re-forms into many mutant species. So, the actual result of irradiation includes destroying what little nutrition remains in already sick food. Then, mutant species of dangerous bacteria are created. Plus, the food is further contaminated with radioactive ions. It is just one more way to make what is currently represented as food even more toxic and defeated, plus, highly dangerous.

The public has been brainwashed into believing that massive food processors and factory farming are the only way to feed the growing population. Yet, it is not working, because the quality of the food is so bad. Well-fed people are happy, peaceful, and productive in every way. Warring nations are not happy, well-balanced societies. Again, taking responsibility to grow gardens, no matter how small, and purchasing from non-chemical local farms are baby steps in the right direction.

It is possible to be totally self-sufficient. A large family in Canada grows all their own food. The growing season is much shorter there, but the food that they produce and gather from the wild is healthy and utterly delicious. The winters are fierce and long, but the root cellar is full of beautiful carrots, potatoes, squash, onions, tomato juice and sauce, green tomato pickles, jarred soups, vegetables, meat, wild berries, nuts, and more. Plus, they produce their own honey. Chicken and eggs are their main protein source. They have no freezer, so the mother cans all their winter food that cannot be stored in the root cellar. Very little is purchased from commercial sources. While this is the ideal way to be self-sustaining, not everyone can do this. However, all efforts to support small non-GMO, non-chemical or organic farmers are also beneficial. The world will thrive, when people work together and help each other to be strong and healthy. Bartering goods and services is becoming quite active again, since the economy has fallen so dramatically.

Changing the way America eats

On the internet Mike Adams is known as the Health Ranger. He has a terrific newsletter called *Natural News*. It is free, and he provides the latest news to help make life better. Anyone can sign up for this excellent information at www.naturalnews.com. Mr. Adams is also quite concerned about the health of American children. Recently, his breaking news was about research published in the journal *BMC Cancer*. Children consume vast quantities of bacon, hot dogs, sausage, ham, and luncheon meats. These same children are 74 percent more likely to contract leukemia than children who abstain from these poisonous processed meats. Besides leukemia, pancreatic cancer and colorectal cancer are also a threat in processed meat consumers. The risk for deadly pancreatic cancer in these meat eaters is 67 percent. This new research once again confirms the link between these cancers and sodium nitrite, the poison in question. These deadly additives are used to make the processed meats more visibly appealing and, supposedly, to increase the shelf life. Dr. Cass Ingram has long been an opponent of sodium nitrite and sodium nitrate. He further discusses all of the dangerous foods, including processed meats, in his book *How to Eat Right and Live Longer*.

As mentioned earlier high fructose corn syrup, a common sweetener found in thousands of foods, is basically made from GMO-tainted corn. That alone is reason to never eat anything containing this substance. Now, Mr. Adams further revealed that new research published in *Environmental Health* confirms that products containing high fructose corn syrup are routinely contaminated with mercury. Apparently, this is not a new occurrence, since seeds have been treated for years with mercurial fungicides. These mercury-laced compounds, such as Ceresan, Semesan, and Panogen, are hazardous not only to the people applying them and the growers themselves, but also they are a long-term poison in the environment. It seems these particular toxic substances are no longer commonly used, but they certainly don't just disappear overnight. At any rate mercury residues are a serious danger to health, especially in children.

What about mercury? Why is it dangerous? Much of the seafood has been contaminated with this noxious material for ages. The dentists even put it in small children's mouths.

Mercury has long been known to be a deadly substance. It is a heavy metal that damages the body especially the brain, lungs, and kidneys. The extent of damage depends upon the type, length, and amount of mercury exposure. The symptoms that arise from this nasty toxin include vision, hearing, and speech impairment, itchy or discolored skin, peripheral neuropathy, edema, and peeling skin. Children commonly exhibit red lips, cheeks, and noses. Loss of hair is usual due to thyroid damage. Also, loss of teeth and nails occur plus increased susceptibility to fungal infections. Kidney problems are rampant, as is profuse sweating. It is not unusual for a child with a mouthful of mercury to experience emotional instability, impaired learning and memory, and insomnia. The list continues, and no doubt, the degree of damage that actually occurs is unknown.

In this day of draconian government regulations and massive persecution/fines for products that cause no harm whatsoever, isn't it strange that certain manufacturers can actually kill people with no restraint or reproof? This means that people must protect themselves. Whether it is danger from vaccinations, dental fillings, contaminated food and water, radiation, or any other harmful exposure, everyone should be aware of what is beneficial for health and what is not. It once was easy to hide the truth, but now anyone who looks for answers can find them.

Another free website which is consumer-minded is www.Mercola.com. These information sites provide the latest input about research, health, and the good, as well as the bad, in the public realm. They are focused on family life and making this country better for all of her people. No one has to agree with everything that is written. However, it is vitally important to use one's God-given ability to think and weigh the benefits and the detriments of all that affects life and liberty. Making an informed decision is your power.

Chapter Six
Food for Fun and Fitness

There are recipes throughout the book that are delicious and wholesome. Experiment and try them all. Use as much non-chemical/organic food as you can find and afford. The quality, flavor, and nutritional difference are worth the extra price. Again, as better food is demanded, better will be available. Then, the prices for organic food will become more competitive. However, keep in mind that organic food is more labor-intensive. Plus, supporting local farmers helps to save shipping costs. Even if the land is in conversion/chemical-free status, it is better than pesticide-laden food found in most stores.

By now it is obvious that good food is mandatory for a healthy and happy life. It has been proven repeatedly that poor food and toxic environmental factors cause an increase in disease. Dr. Weston Price described villages in the Swiss Alps that had no doctors or dentists, because they did not need them. They also had no prisons or insane asylums. The village people worked together, they helped each other, and they lived simple but very balanced, meaningful lives. No food except for sea salt was brought into the communities. No commercial food was ever eaten, and no refined sugar was ever used. All food that they did eat, beef, milk and butter, eggs, honey, whole meal rye bread, garden produce, wild vegetation, and wild berries, kept them in the finest of physical and spiritual balance.

It takes effort to eat well today, but the results are quickly apparent in physical activity and strength as well as mental stability and acuity. The following recipes are full of the vital nutrients that everyone needs. Recently, some friends enjoyed snacking on one of the recipes during a six-hour drive home. The individual had purchased some snacks at a local health food store for her and her family to eat on the trip, but none of the packaged foods were opened. I made the Tomato Flat Bread for them to try. She said they enjoyed it so much, they couldn't leave it alone. The packaged food had no appeal. Hopefully, you will enjoy it as much as they did. It is quite tasty with dips and nut butters, which add even more vitamins, minerals, protein, and fatty acids.

Note: all recipes in this book are highly nutritious. Yet, they are so easy to prepare that most children can make them. They are designed to help people create their own easy, fast, delicious—and most of all—nutritious and healthy recipes.

BREADS AND COOKIES

Tomato Flat Bread

    2 cups organic brown rice flour
    1 cup organic amaranth flour
    1 cup organic teff flour
    ½ cup extra virgin olive oil
    ½ cup chopped sun-dried cherry tomatoes
    ½ cup (soaked) sunflower seeds

1 teaspoon sea salt
2 tablespoons wild oregano/Rhus coriaria mixture
¾ cup water

Combine all ingredients in a large bowl except the water. Add water and gently stir until ingredients are mixed. The mixture should be creamy in texture. Add more water if necessary. Pour onto greased and floured sheet pan. Sprinkle oregano herb and spice mixture (crushed wild oregano with *Rhus coriaria*) on the top and a dusting of fine sea salt for extra flavor. Bake in a 350°F oven for 40 minutes or until lightly browned.

Cinnamon Crunch Bread

2 cups organic brown rice flour
1 cup organic quinoa flour
1 cup organic amaranth flour
½ cup (soaked) sunflower seeds
½ cup chopped pistachios
1 teaspoon sea salt
1 teaspoon cinnamon
2/3 cup cold-pressed sesame oil
1 cup of water
Powdered cinnamon to shake on top of bread

Combine all dry ingredients, plus the sunflower seeds and pistachios, in a large bowl. Gently stir until ingredients are mixed. Add oil and stir until flour is just moistened. Add water and stir just until creamy. Pour the mixture on an oiled and floured sheet pan. Spread mixture to the edges of the pan. Shake extra cinnamon on the top of the bread. Bake in a preheated 350°F oven for about 35 minutes or until lightly browned.

Healthy Peanut Butter Cookies

Peanut butter cookies are still my favorite. Unfortunately, peanuts are a common allergy food for some youngsters. If your child is allergic to peanuts, substitute almond butter, sunflower seed butter, hazelnut butter, Brazil nut butter, hemp seed butter, or pecan butter. These are available in health food stores. They all are delicious. Use almond extract with the almond butter for more flavorful almond cookies. Use organic brown rice flour, because the production of GMO-tainted rice is increasing rapidly. Brown rice flour supplies the much-needed B vitamins.

¾ cup organic crunchy peanut butter
¾ cup raw honey
1 egg
½ cup water or whole milk
2 teaspoons vanilla (almond extract with almond butter)
1 teaspoon sea salt
1 teaspoon baking soda
2 cups organic brown rice flour
1 cup organic spelt or kamut flour

In a large bowl cream honey and nut butter together. Beat egg and combine with water or milk and vanilla (or almond) extract in a small bowl. Add egg mixture to the creamed mixture and stir until smooth. Sift dry ingredients together and add to the nut butter/honey mixture. Gently stir until all dry ingredients are moistened.

Oil and flour a cookie sheet, and drop dough by heaping teaspoonfuls onto the cookie sheet. With the back of a moistened fork, press down lightly on each cookie.

Place cookies in a preheated 350°F oven, and bake for 10 to 12 minutes. When baking with honey, the cookies can burn easily. Therefore, watch them closely and remove as soon as they are golden brown.

Ginger Snappies

1 ¼ cup organic brown rice flour
1 cup teff flour
1 teaspoon ground cinnamon
1 teaspoon ground ginger
½ teaspoon ground cloves
1 teaspoon baking soda
1 teaspoon sea salt
½ cup cold-pressed sesame oil
¼ cup yacon syrup
¼ cup carob molasses
1 teaspoon rice vinegar
½ cup water or organic whole milk
¼ cup pine nuts

Combine all dry ingredients in a large mixing bowl. In another bowl combine the oil, syrup, molasses, vinegar, water or milk, and whip them together. Gently mix the wet ingredients into the dry ones until a dough is formed. Cover the dough and refrigerate for about one hour.

Using a tablespoon drop the dough onto an oiled cookie sheet. Place 3 or 4 pine nuts on the center and press gently with the bottom of an oiled glass so that the cookie is about ½ inch thick. Bake in a preheated 350°F oven for 10 minutes or until golden brown.

This is a good recipe for upset tummies. The ginger makes these cookies a soothing treat, and the yacon, 50% inulin by weight, along with the molasses, creates a healthy snack that is good for everyone. It is plenty sweet without the refined sugar, and it is a nutritious delight.

SOUPS, SALSA, AND SNACKS

Fresh soups—hot and cold

Freshly prepared soup can be so nourishing depending on the ingredients and preparation procedures. Soup is one of my favorite foods, since it provides vitamins, minerals, and many other important food factors to keep the body healthy. It is easy to eat and digest, so even a sickly child benefits greatly from a bowl of luscious soup. It doesn't take a lot of energy to consume.

Soup is commonly a comfort food, especially hot soups during the cold winter evenings and cold soups during the hot summer days. Depending on the ingredients, some vegetables and herbs are warming and some are cooling. Certainly, the whole family will enjoy these delicious recipes and benefit from these fresh wholesome creations no matter what the season.

Summer Sunshine Soup

(For best results use home grown or organic fresh vegetables)

1 large or 2 medium sized ripe tomatoes
1 medium cucumber
1 large green pepper

2 or 3 green onions

1 or more cloves of garlic

1 ounce of honey vinegar or other mild, light-colored vinegar (see www.Americanwildfoods.com)

½ ounce of raw sesame oil

½ ounce of sacha inchi oil or extra virgin olive oil

1 teaspoon sea salt

1 cup tomato juice (optional)

Clean all vegetables thoroughly. If the vegetables are waxed, use a vegetable cleaner to remove it. Then the skin is safe to use as well. Place all ingredients in a food processor or large blender. If you like chunks of vegetables, process/blend in short bursts until it is the consistency you desire. If you want it very soupy, process/blend until all vegetables are liquefied. You may wish to add one cup of tomato juice, if the tomatoes are not totally ripe and juicy. Also, a squeeze of lemon or lime is a tasty addition and adds extra vitamin C.

For a full meal chop carrots, celery, bok choy, parsley, cilantro, Jerusalem artichokes, turnips, and any other vegetable that is preferred, and toss them together. Place about ½ cup of the chopped vegetables in a soup bowl. Pour the cold soup over the chopped vegetables, garnish with chopped greens, and enjoy.

Raw foods, especially when freshly picked, are full of the sun's energy, plus enzymes and flavor that is incomparable.

Cucumber Cooler

3 small to medium cucumbers

3 green onions

1 clove of garlic

    4 cups of full fat organic yogurt
    4 tablespoons fresh dill weed, finely chopped
    1 teaspoon sea salt

Wash, peel, and coarsely chop cucumbers. Wash and coarsely chop green onions. Wash, peel, and smash garlic. Place all ingredients except dill into a food processor or large blender. Process/ blend until smooth. Pour into a large bowl and fold in finely chopped dill. Place in refrigerator until ready to serve.

Hot Winter Soother

    1 large carrot
    1 large potato
    1 stick of celery
    2 cloves of garlic
    1 cup raw peeled and chopped butternut squash
    1 cup organic goat milk or cow's milk; raw milk is best if available
    1 teaspoon sea salt
    ½ teaspoon cumin powder
    ½ teaspoon ground cinnamon
    2 cups filtered water

Put all ingredients (except water) in a food processor or large blender. Process/blend until smooth. Bring the 2 cups of filtered water to a boil. Carefully stir in the boiling water with the vegetable/milk mixture and process/blend until well mixed. This is nice warm soup that must be served and eaten immediately. While you have the pleasure of a warm soup, the enzymes are still intact from the raw vegetables.

Red and Rice Soup

> ½ cup wild rice
> 1½ cups water
> 1 small onion, thinly sliced
> 3 cups of tomato juice
> 1 coarsely chopped carrot
> 1 stick coarsely chopped celery
> 1 cup fresh broccoli tops and peeled stems, chopped
> 1 teaspoon sea salt
> 1 teaspoon oregano herb and spice mixture

Bring water and sea salt to a rapid boil. Add washed and cleaned wild rice and thinly sliced onions to the water. Bring back to a boil, cover, and turn off the heat. Let the rice soak in the water for a minimum of two hours. Repeat the process (bring to a boil, then turn off the heat, and let soak) if the rice is still too hard to eat. Add tomato juice to the rice, when it is tender, and heat just until rice and tomato juice are hot. Add all other ingredients, and heat just until the vegetables are warm. Serve immediately. The vegetables will still be crunchy. The rice will still be whole, but the taste is easily released from the slightly chewy rice. The rice and vegetables hold the heat a little longer than the blender soups, but enjoy it as soon as possible while it is hot.

Creamy Supper Soup

> 3 cups butternut squash
> ½ cup pine nuts
> ½ cup coconut milk
> 1 to 2 cups water

1 teaspoon sea salt
ground cinnamon

Wash the butternut squash, place the whole squash on a baking sheet, and bake in a 350°F oven. Bake until tender or fork easily punctures skin and flesh of the squash. Remove from oven. When the squash is cool enough to easily handle, remove the skin and the seeds from the center. (The seeds are edible when the shells are removed. They are tasty and nutritious.) Place the three cups of squash in the blender with the pine nuts, coconut milk, sea salt, and one cup of water. Blend until mixture is creamy and smooth. Place mixture into a sauce pan, and slowly stir in more water. One or more cups may be needed until desired consistency of soup is achieved. Stir soup until warm. Serve soup with a dusting of ground cinnamon on the top.

SUMMER SALSAS

Some children have very sensitive taste buds, and they prefer very bland foods. Many times their food preferences reflect what the parents choose to eat. However, there are the exceptions, who love the spicy, tangy foods.

The salsas are a spicy food and are normally based upon the Mexican recipes which contain tomato, cumin, and hot peppers. If the taste buds cannot tolerate the caustic peppers, mild ones can be used or even paprika can be used in place of the fiery hot ones. The fiery hot ones can blister the skin, so caution must be used when cooking with them. They are too caustic for small children.

Simply Salsa

3 large, ripe, organic red tomatoes, chopped
1 green pepper, chopped
1 white onion, chopped
1 clove of garlic, smashed and chopped
2 ounces extra virgin olive oil
1 teaspoon powdered cumin
1 teaspoon sea salt
3 tablespoons fresh cilantro, finely chopped (optional)
1 teaspoon oregano spice mixture (crushed wild oregano and Rhus coriaria)
1 hot or mildly hot pepper, finely chopped (optional)

Place extra virgin olive oil in a skillet over medium-low heat. Add chopped white onion and cumin. Gently stir, and as onion begins to become transparent add in garlic, chopped green pepper (hot or mildly hot pepper can also be added), and sea salt. When the green pepper becomes slightly tender, pour off the extra virgin olive oil, and add the chopped tomato. Gently stir all ingredients, including oregano spice mixture, over low heat until warm. Remove from heat, pour into a bowl, add finely chopped cilantro if desired. Salsa is commonly eaten with corn chips. Unfortunately, corn chips are not recommended because of GMO contamination or cross contamination of corn. The various taco/tostada chips are fried in boiling hot grease. Because of the high heat and the continuous use of the oil to fry million of chips, the fat is oxidized. Use salsa with vegetable sticks, bean dishes, or with the Golden American Fries, which is found under Snacks. This recipe is so delicious, and the children will love them. It is made from real potatoes with skin on, so they are highly nutritious and safe to eat.

Eggplant Salsa

1　medium eggplant

¼　cup of sun-dried cherry tomatoes in extra virgin olive oil

¼　cup halved fire-roasted artichoke hearts in extra virgin olive oil

1　clove of garlic

1　teaspoon sea salt

2　teaspoons oregano/Rhus coriaria spice mixture

3　tablespoons capers

Bake the whole eggplant in a 325°F oven until fork penetrates the flesh easily. Let cool. Peel and place in a blender. Add the sun-dried cherry tomatoes and fire roasted artichoke hearts in extra virgin olive oil. Peel, wash, and smash garlic, and place in blender. Add sea salt and oregano spice mixture. Blend until smooth and creamy. Stir in capers and serve as a dip or pesto with vegetables or salad.

SNACKS

I rarely recommend any recipe that requires frying. However, if it is done at a low temperature with organic palm and/or coconut oil, it is quite delicious. So many people eat fried foods on a daily basis, and the fats are usually refined and hydrogenated or partially hydrogenated. These are dangerous fats that cause hardening of the arteries, high blood pressure, high cholesterol, heart attacks, diabetes, skin disorders, and arthritis. That is why today even children have these disorders.

Golden American Fries

>   2 large white potatoes (leave skin on)
>   ½ cup red palm/coconut oil
>   Sea salt

Wash potatoes thoroughly, and cut in half the long way. Cut the long halves into ½ inch fries. Let the fries drain in a colander about 20 minutes and pat dry. Put the oil in a heavy skillet and gently sauté the fries until crispy. They will be beautiful bright golden orange in color. Sprinkle lightly with sea salt and serve immediately. The taste is brilliant. Eat them plain or with the Simply Salsa.

To cook them in the oven, place potatoes on an oiled cookie sheet. Paint on the red palm/coconut oil. Sprinkle sea salt over the fries, and bake in a preheated 350°F oven until crispy and brown.

Bagel Crunchies

>   6 hemp seed bagels (should be stale)
>   ¼ cup sun-dried cherry tomatoes
>   ½ cup extra virgin olive oil (from the sun-dried cherry tomatoes)
>   3 tablespoons minced garlic (optional)
>   2 tablespoons oregano spice mixture (ground wild oregano spice and Rhus coriaria)
>   2 teaspoons fresh basil, finely chopped
>   ½ teaspoon sea salt

Slice the bagels in half. Stand bagels on edges, and thinly slice the bagel halves. There should be 8 to 10 slices per whole bagel. Place slices next to each other on a cookie sheet.

Blend in blender cherry tomatoes, olive oil, garlic, oregano spice, basil, and sea salt. Spread over the bagel slices, and bake in preheated 325°F oven for about 10 to 15 minutes. Turn off oven and let them cool inside the oven. These are delicious hot or cold.

The cherry tomatoes may be omitted. The crisped bagels are also great for nut butter spreads or the salsa.

Sesame Nuts

1 cup English walnuts
1 cup pecans
1 cup sunflower seeds
½ cup raw unhulled sesame seeds
3 tablespoons rice syrup
1 teaspoon sea salt
¼ teaspoon allspice
¼ teaspoon cinnamon

Put the nuts and sunflower seeds in a bowl and cover with water for about five to six hours. Drain off remaining water, and spread them out on a cookie sheet. In a preheated 350°F oven bake the nuts and seeds, stirring occasionally for about 10 minutes or until totally dry and fragrant. Be careful not to burn them.

Spread sesame seeds on a cookie sheet and toast them in a preheated 350°F oven. Stir every five minutes until the seeds are golden. They should have a toasted, buttery flavor.

In a large mixing bowl mix the rice syrup, sea salt, allspice, and cinnamon. Add the hot walnuts, pecans, and sunflower seeds, and stir so that they are evenly coated. Sprinkle the sesame seeds over the nuts and seeds, and gently stir this mixture.

Cover a cookie sheet with oiled paper, or lightly coat with red palm/coconut oil. Spread the nuts and seeds mixture on the cookie sheet to cool.

This recipe will last for up to a week in an airtight container, but around most families it is gone well before then. It is not only delicious, but it is also rich in protein, vitamin E, calcium, iron, B vitamins, and more.

SALADS AND VEGETABLE/FRUIT DISHES

Salads are an easy, tasty, beautiful way to eat live food. In Europe, especially in France, the vegetables for each day's meals are purchased fresh every day from the farmer's market. That means they are picked and eaten in less than 24 hours. Since plant life absorbs the energy from the sun, the sooner it is eaten after picking, the better.

Unfortunately, the vegetables and fruits in the grocery stores in the United States may be weeks—even years—old when you buy it. For example, tomatoes, pineapple, bananas, and avocados are just a few examples of produce that are picked green. Some food is held in cold storage for over a year, and then gassed into what would appear to be a ripened state. Needless to say, the sun's rays are long gone from such "food," and so are the nutrients. We depend on oranges to provided vitamin C. Yet, if they are picked green and are old as well, they will contain none. Much of our food is bulk, useless calories and little else. That's why the United States leads the world in obesity and degenerative illnesses.

Farmer's markets are more common again. Find whatever you can that is as fresh as you can get. Good produce smells wonderful, especially such foods as tomatoes and certain melons. Food should be firm, but not rock hard as the picked-too-green produce is. It shouldn't show signs of deterioration, wilting, or rot. The colors should be bright and fresh. The ideal taste is intense, flavorful, and delicious. Plus, this kind of food nourishes all the cells of the body to make them healthier, and thus, they survive longer. That means better health, less disease, and longer lives free of pain and debilitation. It also means that children will be healthier, happier, smarter, better behaved, and will maintain a better physical condition and appearance.

Eat all sorts of sunshine-soaked salad greens daily and feel the difference. The energy from sunlight plays a major role in nourishing our bodies. The nourished body is stronger, it can be more active, and intelligence is greater.

Try new vegetables and fruits. Some foods one must learn to love, especially when they are new to the palate. So many people are in food ruts, and getting out of ruts can change life for the better.

Sunshine Salad

    1 head fresh organic leaf or romaine lettuce
    1 large red organic tomato, cut into chunks
    1 large yellow organic tomato, cut into chunks
    1 fresh organic green pepper, coarsely chopped
    3 organic asparagus spears, slightly cooked, coarsely chopped
    1 organic sun choke (Jerusalem artichoke) peeled and chopped
    3 Tablespoons (soaked and drained) organic sunflower
       seeds

Wash lettuce carefully and tear into bite-sized pieces. (cutting damages the leaves). Clean all vegetables, and cut or chop into pieces. Lightly toss together all ingredients in a large bowl. Drizzle with dressing just before serving, or allow everyone to add their own. Leftover salad may be kept for the next meal if it does not have dressing on it. Sunflower seeds are even more nutritious and easier to digest when soaked. Place ½ cup of sunflower seeds in a bowl and cover with filtered or clean bottled water. Soak overnight or at least for five or six hours. This will begin the sprouting process. Then drain any excess water, and sprinkle sea salt over the seeds. They can be used immediately or stored covered in the refrigerator and used as needed.

Sunshine Dressing

½ cup Styrian pumpkinseed oil
2 tablespoons cold-pressed sesame oil
1 tablespoon cold-pressed black seed oil
1 tablespoon sacha inchi oil
½ cup honey vinegar
1 teaspoon Hungarian paprika
1 teaspoon yellow mustard
1 teaspoon raw honey
1 teaspoon sea salt
  freshly ground black pepper to taste

Combine all ingredients and blend in a blender. Pour immediately over salad, or put into a shaker bottle. Shake well before dressing the salad. This dressing is even better when it marinates overnight. The oils in this dressing provide chlorophyll, vitamin E, essential fatty acids, amino acids, and more.

Potato Delight

Small, young food is tender, tasty, and full of life. Small red potatoes with the skin on baked just until slightly soft are perfect for any potato salad. The nourishment is in the skin.

8 or 10 small-to-medium red potatoes (the skin should not show any tinges of green, and they must be well washed with eyes removed)

1 large organic red tomato, chopped, or 10 cherry tomatoes, halved

1 stick of celery, chopped

2 small carrots, chopped

1 small green pepper, chopped

6 roasted artichoke hearts, chopped

3 red radishes, chopped

2 green onions, chopped

3 tablespoons fresh dill, chopped

¼ cup pine nuts

Prepare the potatoes and bake them in a 350°F oven. Clean and chop vegetables. When potatoes are cooled and chopped, add all other chopped vegetables and pine nuts. Pour over dressing and lightly stir until well mixed.

Potato Delight Dressing

¼ cup extra virgin olive oil (from roasted artichokes)

2 tablespoons sesame oil

2 tablespoons Styrian pumpkinseed oil

¼ cup mild vinegar (apple cider or honey vinegar)

1 teaspoon sea salt

1   clove garlic, smashed and chopped or use garlic press
    (optional)

Combine all ingredients in a small blender, and blend until all ingredients are well mixed. Pour over potato salad. This is a good dressing for other vegetable salads as well.

White and Green Salad

6 to 8 leaves of bok choy
2 cups Chinese cabbage
1 cup of broccoli sprouts
3 tablespoons parsley
3 tablespoons dill

Wash all greens carefully, because they can be contaminated with parasites and pathogens such as E. coli. The commercial pickers who handle the plants many times do not have sanitation facilities to wash their hands after defecating. Even the so called pre-washed salad material should be rinsed in cold water. Loss of health is not worth the few extra minutes it takes to properly clean food before it is eaten, especially raw food.

Bok choy is an interesting and tasty, crunchy salad green. Also, it is frequently used in stir frying. There is a minimum of green leafy material, so tear that part into bite-sized pieces. Then cut the white stem part into ½ inch slices. Chinese cabbage should be finely sliced to a slaw-like consistency. Make it as fine as you can. Some food processors will do the job, or just use a long knife. Broccoli sprouts after washing need to be thoroughly drained, the tiny plants separated, and placed in the bowl with the greens. Prepare three tablespoons each of finely chopped parsley and dill. Mix all ingredients together lightly with clean hands. This is a light and airy salad with an interesting combination of flavors. This salad contains vitamin C and folic acid, plus minerals.

Creamy Dreamy Dressing

    1 avocado
    1 medium tomato
    1 green onion
    1 clove of garlic (optional)
    1 teaspoon sea salt
    2 ounces of honey vinegar or white balsamic vinegar
    2 ounces of extra virgin olive oil

Clean vegetables, peel avocado, tomato, and garlic, and cut the root end off the green onion. Cut all vegetables into chunks, and place them into a blender along with sea salt, vinegar and olive oil. Blend until creamy. Put into serving bowl with spoon to dress the White and Greens Salad. This is also quite a good dip for vegetables such as carrot sticks, celery, cauliflower, and broccoli. If the dressing is too thick, it may be thinned with lemon or lime juice.

VEGETABLE AND FRUIT DISHES

For small children raw fruit can be finely grated and mixed with mashed avocado and a bit of raw honey or yacon syrup. Any fruit or non-starchy vegetable may be used. Even young children have food preferences. If they experience adverse symptoms after eating, it may well be an allergic reaction.

Children have many more reactions than ever before, because their small systems cannot tolerate the over 9000 chemicals, toxins, and the GMOs that adulterate food today. That is why using organic foods and homegrown foods that are as fresh as possible are the best choices.

Baby food is so easy to make that it is actually silly to buy jarred food. When it is purchased, the food is months or years old. Unless it is organic with no additives and preservatives, no one can be sure what is in it. Also, jarred food is more expensive than making baby food from fresh food. The following are baby food suggestions that people for generations have used successfully.

Fruit is the first food for babies, because it is easiest to digest. Then, meat is usually the next food to add. Some vegetables are easier to tolerate than others. Starchy grains, beans, and certain vegetables are difficult if not impossible for the baby to digest. Unfortunately, cereals are usually the first food many babies receive. Before a child has teeth, there is virtually little to no starch splitting enzyme present for the digestion of starchy foods. Thus, digestive disorders are common. Dr. Melvin Page and Dr. J. H. Tilden adamantly agreed that children are not capable of eating starchy foods until two or even three years of age. By this time they have a full set of teeth, can chew their food, and are producing ptyalin in their saliva. This enzyme combines with food via saliva while chewing and breaks down starch into a digestible sugar.

Always wash all food carefully, when preparing baby food. The tiny blenders are so fast and easy to use and clean. They make food preparation of any kind so fast and an absolute joy. The baby's palate does not require seasoning and definitely not refined sugar or corn syrup. It is shocking to see people turning their children into sugar addicts, while they are still babies. When parents are addicted, it seems to them that feeding the child sugar is fun, a treat, or a kindness. Actually, it leads to the greatest kinds of misery: both obesity and diabetes and even cancer.

FIRST FOOD FOR BABIES

Dr. Melvin Page's extensive worldwide research confirmed that a baby should continue to nurse *healthy* mother's milk until all teeth have developed. That is why mothers must eat healthy food for the proper development of their children and for their own health and wellness. Ideally, the first year of life babies' food should be exclusively mothers' milk.

The following fruit are best for baby's first solid food.

The baby can be fed all fruit with a small baby spoon.

- Mashed dates, figs, prunes, and raisins: thin with water so that it is easier for baby to learn to eat and swallow.
- Ripe bananas: they can be mashed and fed with a spoon or given to the baby as finger food.
- Avocado, raw and mashed.
- Unsweetened applesauce or grated raw apple without the skin
- Apricots, cook in a small amount of water just until tender. Blend until smooth. Use dried or raw apricots.
- Grated fresh pear

When the fruit is fresh and raw only prepare the amount the child will eat at one sitting.

First foods for chewing

When children can adequately chew, they can begin eating shredded vegetables and chopped fruit by themselves. The following are some recipes for the young, but they are so delicious everyone can enjoy them.

Kiddie Slaw
_____

¼ head of organic green cabbage
1 organic carrot
½ red apple
½ green pear
a half lemon or orange

Finely grate the cabbage and carrot separately. Then grate the apple and pear separately. All ingredients can be combined or remain separate but eaten together. Arrange small scoops in a bowl and garnish with raisins that have been soaked in warm water. A squeeze or two of orange and lemon juice over the grated apple and pear will keep them from turning brown. The citrus juice stops the oxidation process.

Chopped Veggie Surprise
_____

This is a great salad for children who are constipated, a common problem today.

1 small to medium organic cucumber, finely chopped
1 medium organic carrot, finely chopped
1 stick organic celery, finely chopped
3 stewed prunes

Clean and chop vegetables individually in a blender or food processor. Stir all blended vegetables gently together with chopped prunes. For older children add soaked sunflower seeds for additional protein and B vitamins.

Cottage Salad

- ¼ cup finely chopped organic spinach
- ¼ cup grated organic carrot
- 2 cups full fat organic cottage cheese
- 2 leaves of organic romaine lettuce

Wash spinach carefully, because it may contain grit and sand. With a sharp knife finely chop spinach by hand. Grate carrot with grater. Add spinach and carrot to cottage cheese. Serve over shredded romaine lettuce. There are some tasty season salts that can be added to the cottage cheese mixture. Also, fresh herbs contain so many important nutrients that it is an added benefit to include finely chopped parsley and dill weed or basil.

Broccoli Slaw

- 3 or 4 organic broccoli stems, peeled
- 2 organic medium carrots
- 2 organic celery sticks

Wash and peel broccoli stems and grate. Clean carrots and grate. Wash and remove strings from celery and grate. Combine all ingredients and garnish with soaked raisins. **Quick and Easy Soup:** This vegetable mixture can be added to 2 cups of chicken broth or vegetable broth and heated just until hot. Be sure to add 1 teaspoon of sea salt, since vegetables are so high in potassium.

Nut 'n Chicken Salad

   2 cups organic chicken breast, cubed
   ½ cup chopped organic celery
   ½ cup chopped fresh organic pineapple
   ½ cup fresh organic grapes, halved and seeded
   ½ cup coarsely chopped pecans or other nuts as desired
   2 tablespoons finely chopped organic parsley
   4 tablespoons honey vinegar or rice vinegar
   4 tablespoons raw organic sesame oil or extra virgin olive oil
   1 teaspoon stone ground mustard
   sea salt to taste

Combine the first 6 ingredients in a mixing bowl. Mix the vinegar, oil, mustard, and sea salt together and pour over salad mixture. Mix together lightly.

Fresh Kiddie Lunches

   1 or 2 chopped raw prunes
   1 or 2 slices raw goat cheese
   1 small tomato, diced
   1 romaine lettuce leaf, shredded

Arrange tomato on shredded lettuce and chopped prunes on cheese on a small luncheon plate.

½ fresh peach, coarsely chopped
1 slice cantaloupe, coarsely chopped
1 serving grapes without stems or seeds
1 slice soft goat or sheep cheese
1 lettuce leaf

Arrange all of the above ingredients on lettuce leaf.

4 ripe, organic strawberries, quartered
¼ cup organic blueberries
½ cup full-fat organic cottage cheese

Arrange attractively on small plate.

8 or 10 fresh, organic spinach leaves
4 large organic strawberries, cut into halves
2 tablespoons pine nuts
1 ounce of fresh lemon juice
1 ounce of fresh, raw honey
1 tablespoon Styrian pumpkinseed oil

On a small plate arrange spinach, strawberries and pine nuts. Combine lemon juice, raw honey, and pumpkinseed oil and drizzle over salad.

All of the lunches may include a small rice cake or rice cracker with organic nut butter of the child's choice. Besides peanut butter, there are a variety of nut butters such as almond, pecan, Brazil nut, walnut, sunflower seed, and macadamia nut.

Raw Nut Butter: It is easy to make in a blender. Place one cup of fresh, raw nuts into a blender and blend. Slowly add while blending about ¼ cup of raw sesame oil, depending on desired consistency. (Extra virgin olive oil or nut oils can be used in place of sesame oil.) Coarsely chop another ¼ cup of nuts and add to the creamy nut mixture, if crunchy style nut butter is preferred.

Super Balls

8 oz. organic dried unsulfured apricots
8 oz. organic golden raisins
1 cup soaked almonds, dried in the oven
½ tsp. sea salt
¼ cup unhulled sesame seeds

Using a food processor finely chop all ingredients in order: apricots, then raisins, then almonds, and sesame seeds. Place all chopped ingredients in a bowl and add sea salt. Mix with hands and roll into balls. They can be rolled in carob powder, lucuma powder, or finely chopped coconut. Store in a covered container in the refrigerator.

Healthy Fruit and Nut Bars

1 cup dried organic figs
1 cup dried organic dates

   1 cup seedless organic raisins
   ¼ cup pecans
   ¼ cup organic sunflower seeds
   ¼ cup pistachios
   1 teaspoon sea salt

Place dried fruit in a food processor and blend until smooth. Place the fruit mixture into a mixing bowl. Stir in chopped nuts and salt, and form into balls. Roll balls in shredded, unsweetened coconut if desired. Or roll in lucuma powder, which is also tasty and full of nutrients.

Note: Sunflower seeds should always be organic. This is because a caustic herbicide is used to kill the flowering plants, so they can dry and be harvested more quickly.

Hawaiian Pineapple Delight

   1 small pineapple
   2 ounces ground fresh pistachios
   2 ounces grated coconut

Peel and core golden ripe pineapple. Chop pineapple, and combine with the ground fresh pistachios and grated coconut. To serve use a platter covered with large fresh green leaves. Serve the chopped pineapple nut mixture garnished with fresh strawberries. Note: Any leftover fruit can be put into blender with tangerine juice or orange juice and ice. This is delicious with a nutritious rice bran breakfast supplement powder.

Date Boats

    12 large dates, cut in half
    ½ cup nut butter: pecan, peanut, or almond

Spread nut butter on each date half. Arrange on a plate, cover, and place in the refrigerator. Chill for at least one hour.

Creamy Date Boats

    12 large dates, cut in half
    ½ cup organic cream cheese
    ½ cup nut butter: pecan, peanut, or almond
    2   tablespoons chopped pistachios

Spread cream cheese on each date half. Carefully spread a layer of nut butter on cream cheese. Garnish with chopped pistachios. Arrange on a plate, cover, and place in the refrigerator. Chill for at least one hour.

Banana Ice Cream

    3 ripe bananas
    ¼ cup organic whole milk

Place bananas in a freezer. Bananas should be ripe, but no brown spots. Freeze until solid. Remove skin, and cut into one inch pieces. Place banana in a blender, and add the milk a little at a time. Use only enough milk to make it creamy. For a special dessert layer banana ice cream in parfait dishes and alternate layers with whipped cream. Top with chopped nuts.

Whipped Cream Topping

    1 pint organic whipping cream
    1 teaspoon vanilla
    3 tablespoons golden berry syrup or yacon syrup

Place whipping cream in a chilled bowl. Whip with a wire whip or mixer until cream holds a peak. Then add vanilla and syrup. Whip again just until mixed.

MAIN DISHES

Dishes made simply with organic ingredients are easy and provide much nourishment. Using a wide variety of foods creates more opportunity for a wider variety of nutrients. A child should eat a combination of raw and cooked foods. Some foods need to be slightly steamed to destroy the spicules or other natural components which inhibit digestion. Of course, breads are baked, but some recipes are prepared in a dehydrator. The low heat keeps important enzymes from being lost.

Speaking of a wide variety of foods available today, even organic pizza crusts are available in health food stores. Some are made with whole grains and without the refined oils. They are an excellent base for a fast meal that kids love.

Fat is a necessary component in the diet, and some fats and oils are preferable to others in food preparation. Canola oil, corn oil, and soy oil are not recommended for daily use. Neither is eating foods prepared with margarine and hydrogenated or partially hydrogenated oils. Not only are they mainly produced from genetically engineered crops, but the refining processes are detrimental. Even safflower and sunflower seed oils are undesirable, since they are high in polyunsaturates (omega-6s) with no omega-3s to balance them.

Butter is always the best choice over margarine of any kind. Organic spring butter is the most nutritious and beneficial of all fats, since it is rich in vitamins A and D.

The best cooking and baking oils are extra virgin olive oil, red palm oil/coconut oil, butter or ghee, and cold-pressed sesame and peanut oils. The Styrian pumpkinseed oil and sacha inchi oil are superb for making salad dressings. However, they must be consumed if the benefits they provide are enjoyed. (don't leave in the bottom of the bowl.) These oils are also an excellent addition to smoothies due to their essential fatty acid composition. Pumpkinseed oil is very high in vitamin E, chlorophyll, and phytosterols. The phytosterols in Styrian pumpkinseed oil are beneficial for the hormone system. Sacha inchi is a major source of omega-3 fatty acids and vitamin E. This oil is 54% omega-3s by weight, making it the richest known source. It is a good source of beta carotene and amino acids. No other omega-3 oil provides these significant amino acids. The additional amino acids are important for vegetarians and especially vegans. It's important to remember that neither of these oils should be used for frying or baking.

Nourishment should always be the main focus when eating. However, we have become a society focused on self indulgence and mere pleasure. As a result disease is rampant. Children have more killer diseases than ever before. The United States ranks among the highest in infant mortality, as high as many third world countries. Chronic illness, sudden death, and physical and mental abnormalities are the norm rather than the unusual. Providing beautiful food, a higher level of spiritual awareness, and a loving environment can completely change all of that. Now, let's move on to the main course dishes.

Total Temptation Stir-Fry

¼ cup red palm/coconut oil

1 medium onion, chopped into bite-sized pieces

1 organic green pepper, chopped into bite-sized pieces

½ lb. buffalo or elk sirloin, cut into bite-sized pieces (use free range or organic beef if buffalo or elk are unavailable)

1 organic red pepper, chopped into bite-sized pieces

1 to 3 cloves garlic, smashed and chopped (optional)

1 cup of bean sprouts

1 cup broccoli, chopped

1 cup cauliflower pieces, chopped

¼ cup sunflower seeds, soaked, drained and dried

2 tablespoons toasted sesame seeds

1 teaspoon sea salt

After washing and chopping all vegetables, let them thoroughly drain in a colander or pat dry. In a large skillet melt red palm/coconut oil until hot, but not smoking. Add chopped onions and meat. Cook until lightly browned. Add the remaining ingredients, and cook just until the color of the vegetables brightens and they are tender, but still crunchy. Remove from heat, and serve over organic brown rice. For vegetarian and vegans merely leave out the meat, but add nuts and seeds, such as organic walnuts, black seed, and pine nuts.

Brown Rice

Prepare the rice before the stir-fry.

2 cups organic brown rice, rinsed and cleaned

½ cup wild rice, rinsed and cleaned

3 cups water

2 organic vegetable/herbal seasoning cubes
1 teaspoon sea salt

Bring water to a boil. Add washed brown and wild rice to the boiling water. Add sea salt and vegetable/herbal seasoning cubes, and let the cubes dissolve in the water. Stir the rice to mix the seasoning evenly. Bring the water back to a boil, cover the pan, and turn off the heat. Let this rice mixture remain covered, and check consistency of the rice in a few hours. (This process may be done at bedtime, and the rice can then soak over night.) If it has not totally absorbed all the liquid and is still too crunchy, add water if needed, and bring the mixture back to a boil. Let it stand for at least one more hour. Heat the rice, while stir fry is cooking. Serve as a side dish, or place a heaping mound on a plate and top with the colorful stir fry.

RICE REMAINDERS

I always make extra rice. There are so many things you can do with it as a hot main dish, hot side dish, or a cold salad. The following are some yummy ideas. Make up your own recipes too.

Place leftover rice (at least two cups, cooked) in a skillet with three tablespoons hot red palm/coconut oil, and add leftover diced organic turkey or chicken and chopped vegetables. Use chopped green beans, asparagus, cherry tomatoes, leeks, parsley, dill, carrots or whatever combination that is available. Add up to one cup of cooked beans, peas, or lentils if desired. For some people beans cause allergy or digestive problems. Stir gently until completely mixed. If you over stir, it becomes a gummy mess. Combine a package of dried organic mushroom soup or onion soup and ¾ cup of water. Mix until dry ingredients are dissolved. Pour soup evenly over rice mixture. Cook over low temperature until hot and rice begins to absorb soup mixture. For vegetarians and vegans leave out the turkey and chicken and continue with the recipe. Add nuts and seeds to increase the protein, vitamins, and minerals.

It is ideal to make this salad with wild rice alone, but it is also delicious with a combination of different types of rice. Place three cups of cooked rice in large bowl. Add six to eight chopped, roasted artichoke hearts (they come in extra virgin olive oil), ½ cup halved cherry tomatoes (fresh or sun-dried cherry tomatoes in extra virgin olive oil), four green onions chopped, ¼ cup chopped pecans and/or sunflower seeds, two tablespoons capers, ¼ cup raw Jerusalem artichokes or turnips chopped, 1 teaspoon sea salt, and three tablespoons finely chopped parsley and dill weed. Add ¼ cup extra virgin olive oil. Use the oil from the artichoke hearts or the cherry tomatoes for extra flavor. Then add three ounces of honey vinegar or a good balsamic vinegar. Gently stir all ingredients until coated with vinegar and oil. Serve as side dish or as a main dish over lettuce.

Organic brown or basmati rice is preferable for this dish. With fruit it is a little sweeter and lighter. Place three cups of cooked rice in a large mixing bowl. Peel and section a large orange, cut into bite-sized pieces, and add to the rice. The rest of the fruit will be whatever is in season. For example, add to cooked rice raw organic (washed) fresh fruit such as one cup of fresh cherries, pitted and cut into halves; one peach or nectarine, peeled, seeds removed, and cut into bite-sized pieces; two apricots, peeled, seeds removed, and cut into bite-sized pieces; one cup of red and green grapes, cut into halves, and seeds removed; one kiwi fruit, peeled and cut into bite-sized pieces, ½ cup blueberries; ½ cup of strawberries, stemmed, and cut into halves; ½ cup pine nuts; and ½ cup of pineapple, peeled, cored, and cut into bite-sized pieces. Mix ½ cup of cream, ½ cup of raw milk, two tablespoons of raw honey, two tablespoons of raw yacon syrup, and 10 drops of cinnamon oil and mix well. Pour over rice and fruit mixture. Eat immediately or leave out the pineapple. It will degrade the cream dressing. You can also use the almond or hazelnut amazake, a fermented rice drink for a dressing, if no dairy is desired. Then, no additional sweetener is required. This is a lovely dessert or even a main dish for lunch.

Spanish rice is usually loved by one and all. Years ago I learned to make it with bacon. Since bacon is a nitrated meat, it should not be used. This is also a delicious way to enjoy rice. In a large skillet combine ½ cup of chopped green pepper, ½ cup of chopped onion, ½ cup chopped smoked organic turkey, three cloves of smashed and finely chopped garlic (optional), and a mild or hot pepper finely chopped with no seeds (optional), and sauté in three ounces of sesame oil. Cook until onions are clear and green pepper is tender.

Add to the skillet two cups of organic, cooked brown rice, one medium-sized can of organic tomato sauce, ½ cup of sliced black olives, one teaspoon of sea salt, and one teaspoon of toasted sesame seeds. Carefully stir until all ingredients are mixed and covered with tomato sauce. Cook just until hot. Serve immediately as a side dish or as a main course. Garnish with grated raw goat or sheep cheese.

Pizza Prize

> 1 prepared organic pizza crust
> 1 can of organic pizza sauce
> ¼ cup crumbled organic feta cheese
> ½ cup finely chopped organic onion
> ½ cup finely chopped organic green pepper
> ¼ cup chopped green olives
> ¼ cup grated organic mozzarella cheese
> 3 tablespoons oregano herb and spice mixture (crushed oregano and Rhus coriaria)
> ¼ cup chopped black olives

Spread pizza sauce evenly over the thawed pizza crust. Evenly distribute onion, green peppers, green olives, black olives, and oregano spice on top of the pizza crust. On one side of the pizza sprinkle the grated mozzarella cheese, and sprinkle the crumbled feta on the other side. Bake in a preheated 425°F oven until crust is done and cheese is melted. Enjoy a healthy pizza fresh out of the oven with a green salad.

Oven-baked Veggies with Greek Super Sauce

> 4 red potatoes cut into large cubes, skin on

  1 medium sweet potato, peeled and cut into large cubes
  1 large or 2 medium-sized parsnips, scraped and cut into
     bite-sized chunks
  2 medium carrots cut into large chunks
  1 small eggplant, peeled, cut into large cubes
  3 small onions, quartered
 10 sun-dried cherry tomatoes, cut into halves
  6 roasted artichoke hearts, cut into halves
  1 head of garlic, all cloves peeled
  ½ cup toasted pecans
  ½ cup of extra virgin olive oil
  ½ cup sesame oil
  5 drops of cumin oil in extra virgin olive oil
  2 teaspoons coarse sea salt

Clean and prepare all vegetables by cutting them into cubes or pieces. Leave the garlic cloves whole. The eggplant should be soaked in one cup of water with one teaspoon of sea salt dissolved in the water for one hour. Remove and let drain. Place vegetables and pecans in a large bowl. Mix the extra virgin olive oil (use the extra virgin olive oil from the roasted artichoke hearts and the sun-dried cherry tomatoes, since it is already beautifully flavored), the sesame oil, and the cumin oil. Pour over vegetables and marinate for one hour. Preheat the oven to 350°F, and place vegetables on a cookie sheet. Sprinkle coarse sea salt over vegetables. Bake for 30 minutes, and stir as needed to ensure even browning. Check to see if vegetables are just tender but not overcooked. Serve with goat's cheese or lamb chops. Use with Spicy Cream Sauce in the following recipe.

Spicy Cream Sauce

> The surprise here is this recipe contains no dairy.
> 2 small to medium eggplants
> 1 or 2 garlic cloves (optional)
> 2 green onions
> 1 large red ripe tomato
> 1 small green pepper
> 1 teaspoon sea salt
> 2 tablespoon wild oregano spice (wild crushed oregano and Rhus coriaria)
> 3 tablespoons sesame oil
> 3 tablespoons apple cider vinegar
> ¼ cup pine nuts

Wash eggplants. Bake whole in a 350°F oven until fork easily punctures the flesh. Remove them from the oven and let them cool to room temperature. Clean and peel raw garlic. (Garlic can be baked in its skin with eggplants for a milder taste) Clean and remove root base from green onions and cut each of them into four pieces. Wash and core tomato. When eggplants are cool, peel and cut them into large pieces, and put into blender. (If the garlic was also baked, peel it and add to the blender) If using raw garlic, smash it with the flat side of a heavy knife to release the flavor, and add to blender with green onion pieces, the tomato halved, sea salt, sesame oil, apple cider vinegar, and oregano spice. Blend until smooth and creamy. Coarsely chop pine nuts, and stir into blended mixture. Use immediately with meat and vegetable dishes as a sauce. After refrigeration it becomes more like a spread and can be used with crackers or bread and vegetable sticks.

Surprise Package Stew

   6   organic ground meat patties or 6 veggie burgers
   (1/3 organic ground beef, 1/3 organic ground lamb, and
   1/3 organic ground turkey, ½ pound of each)
   6   unpeeled red potatoes
   6   carrots
   6   celery sticks
   1   large onion, chopped
   6   pats of butter
   sea salt to taste
   curry powder (optional)
   ½ cup grated, raw goat cheese

Tear off six sheets of foil, about 12 inches square. Combine the three types of ground meat, and form six patties. Slice a red potato onto each sheet of foil. Place a patty (meat or veggie) on top of the potato slices. Add a sliced carrot, a chopped celery stick, and some chopped onion on top of each meat or veggie patty. Place a pat of butter on top of each, and season with sea salt and curry powder. Carefully seal each packet and place sealed side up on a baking sheet. Bake in a preheated 350°F oven for 30 to 40 minutes. Place packets on plates, and pierce the foil to let the steam out. Let everyone open their packages, and add grated cheese if desired.

Festive Brunch Eggs

   1 ½ lbs. organic ground round
   2 tablespoons extra virgin olive oil
   2 large organic onions, chopped

3 cloves, minced garlic
½ lb. fresh organic spinach, kale, or collards, chopped
½ lb. shiitake mushrooms
1½ teaspoon sea salt
1 teaspoon wild oregano
½ cup organic red pepper, chopped
6 organic eggs, beaten
½ cup raw goat or sheep milk cheese, grated

In a large skillet brown the meat, onions, and garlic in extra virgin olive oil. Gently stir mixture, and cook until onions are clear. Greens should be washed to remove any sand or dirt. They must be well drained, and chopped. Add greens, mushrooms, and seasoning to meat mixture. Cook just until greens are softened and bright in color. Over low heat add egg mixture, and stir to combine all ingredients. When eggs are set, the dish is ready to place in a serving bowl. Garnish with grated cheese.

This next dish is a tasty meatless meal. It is rich in calcium and is especially good for children, who need this calming nutrient.

Green Wisdom

1 cup organic spinach, chopped
1 cup organic kale, chopped
1 cup organic collard greens, chopped
½ cup organic onion, chopped
½ cup organic red bell pepper, chopped
½ cup mushrooms, chopped
½ cup pine nuts

1 tablespoon organic sesame seeds
½ cup water
1 cube vegetable seasoning

Wash all of the greens carefully, and coarsely chop them. Dissolve the vegetable seasoning cube in the water in a large skillet. Add the greens and remaining ingredients, except pine nuts and sesame seeds. While gently stirring, cook over medium heat, just until the vegetables are tender and easy to chew. Add pine nuts and sesame seeds to mixture and serve immediately.

Spaghetti Surprise in 5 Minutes

What is the surprise? There is no wheat in this fast recipe, no grains at all. Then what is it that resembles a well-known spaghetti noodle? Read on and enjoy this recipe.

1 long green zucchini
1 jar organic tomato spaghetti sauce, unsweetened
½ lb. ground round, beef or lamb
1 medium onion, chopped
½ cup crumbled goat cheese
¼ cup extra virgin olive oil

Some food processors will make long zucchini "noodles." Otherwise, cut the peeled zucchini in half lengthwise. Keep cutting length-wise until long strands of "spaghetti" are formed. In a sauce pan heat the spaghetti sauce. For meat eaters: in a small skillet brown the meat and onion. Add the sautéed meat and onion to the heated sauce.

Drizzle "noodles" with extra virgin olive oil and place in 350°F oven to heat. When noodles and sauce are hot, place noodles on plates, pour sauce over, and garnish with crumbled goat cheese. Surround with fresh, raw salad greens.

Have fun with the recipes, and enjoy them. Don't be afraid to alter them to your liking. Most of the recipes are so easy that children can help with the preparation as well. Plus, these dishes provide dense nutrition for the whole family.

Chapter Seven
Conclusion

Children are our most important commodity. They are the hope for the future of the entire world. However, their health is being systematically destroyed. Foul air filled with noxious chemicals and depleted uranium, water contaminated with deadly chemicals and pharmaceutical drugs: all are a part of the destruction. The irreversible changing of the genetic structure of natural plant life with the addition of foreign bodies, such as viruses and bacteria, is causing further destruction. Insect and animal matter is shot randomly into the genes of plant life to be forever altered. That is the GMOs. If this isn't enough, hundreds of chemicals are added to genetically modified foods, which are then further refined and devitalized. Plus, in processed food some 9,000 noxious chemicals are used. The result is food which is entirely different than the original sources designed by our creator. No restrictions are placed upon those who are damaging the most important resources in the world. These resources are not minerals, crops, or jewels but, rather, our children. This downward spiral can only be halted by individual effort and, ultimately, all people coming together for the greater good.

Children adapt to their surroundings. They soon learn to identify certain flavors and smells as being their comfort foods. They quickly become programmed and addicted to sugar and chocolate, hot grease and fried foods, chemically-tainted drinks, and all things artificial. Nourishment is never a consideration. The resulting diseases of civilization, such as diabetes, ADD, ADHD, asthma, Crohn's disease, multiple sclerosis, and even cancer, are treated as the world's greatest mysteries. This is total proven nonsense, and the children are paying a terrible price for living in a supposedly sophisticated society that will ultimately lead to the destruction of the human race. Every generation is further corrupted and weakened.

There is no doubt that a poor diet corrupts the physical well-being. Obesity and degenerative disease are rampant and will remain so until better nutritional choices are made individually and collectively. However, it is not just the physical structure that is corrupted. Poor nutrition creates the "difficult" child. It also creates the "depressed" child as well as adult. Negative emotions are also a part of the package, since the brain cannot function adequately without appropriate nourishment. These GMO/refined/fast food options only lead to physical illness, mental deficiencies, and a corruption of the ethics and soul. A well-fed society suffers from few diseases and physical debilities. The people of such a society are productive to the highest degree. They care about all fellow humans. They are happy, joyful and able to live in a state of love and human goodness—people like the Hunzans.

The divine creator designed everything on this planet in the greatest perfection. Humans are allowed the gift of free choice. This means that every individual can think and do whatever he/she wants within certain boundaries. If the choice is made to follow the enlightened path, the highest and finest purposes are sought. That affects every choice made. Needless to say, this includes the food and drinks that are consumed, because overall health depends on those selections. The books that are read reflect the growth of the mind and the increase of knowledge and wisdom. Beautiful music can lift the soul with its high vibration. Reflection on where life's path is leading and the true purpose of every individual soul helps to maintain the sense of urgency to do all that can be done on this short journey on planet earth. This planet and humanity are on a parallel. If the planet is exploited with reckless abandon, it cannot support the lives of the human population. Even little children should know that if they spend their entire allowance as soon as it is received, there is nothing left for future needs. This doesn't take advanced degrees to understand.

It is apparent that government has no concern for the rights of humanity. The government is supposed to serve the people. Instead, it has become the master. Yet, none of it really matters. The thoughts of every individual are the power. What people do collectively makes the difference. It starts with the power of one. That one is you. Choose to make a difference, and it will happen. Above all never worry. Keep your heart, mind, eyes, and soul on all that is positive and productive. Unconditional love must be the focus. When decisions are made from the basis of unconditional love, there can be no bad decisions.

Civilizations crumble when the material world, wealth, and power for the few are the only focus. Universal growth and unity occur, when a higher power is always remembered with gratitude and overwhelming love. Those sick in mind, body and soul need help and prayers.

When a person is ill, there are many reasonable ways to make the body better. Yet, if the soul is ignored, perfect health will not be achieved. It is like being chronically ill, when the light of the highest power is not part of the prescription. Children need to know that there is an almighty power that governs the entire universe. This almighty being protects us and cares for us. Therefore, there is no need for fear. Only that supreme power is totally just and righteous. Every person comes to this planet to grow, learn, and, ideally, reach a higher level. All souls are at different levels. Parental responsibility is to protect and guide each soul that has been put into the family unit. However, ultimately, everyone is responsible to fulfill his/her own purpose.

Larson discusses in his book *Why We Are What We Are* that how a child is nourished both physically and mentally, will determine the development of either the anterior or posterior pituitary. There are several major factors that positively affect the pituitary. This includes good healthy food and drink, literature and material that expedite the brain's ability to think in a higher realm, and beautiful music. All of these together increase the size of the anterior pituitary. This individual continues to seek a higher path for a lifetime.

Even the thinking of destructive thoughts is dangerous. For instance, according to Larson when human prurient desires are the focus, the posterior pituitary over develops and enlarges. This is the master gland, and so any disruption of it will have a major impact on the whole body. Lower priorities, including poor food choices, sexual aberrations, pornography, alcohol and drug abuse, loud and raucous music will be the choices. When this occurs, the individual will fail to follow the path of light. This will be to such a degree that he/she will often become a failure for most positive activities. This person may even adopt criminal behavior. Thus, the physical body is affected by the chosen spiritual path or lack of it.

A child must be free to develop the soul that he/she is, but parents are his/her guides and mentors. Every child in the family needs assistance to learn to make healthy choices. Again, this must begin with the best food selections. They must learn that it is important to have friends who are fine and true. It is a desirable focus to learn whatever expands the mind, and, thus, to develop in a superior way. It should be a goal for the entire family to develop individual talents and skills. The finest path is to seek to achieve all things, which lift the soul to a higher level of existence. This is a huge responsibility, yet few realize what a commitment raising a child really is. If a flower grows in a garden of weeds, it will soon be overwhelmed. Children left to their own devices seldom reach their highest capabilities. Nor without guidance can they nourish their bodies. Nor can they behave appropriately unless they are properly nourished mentally and physically.

Most oriental societies have always cherished their children. They believe that children are the greatest family treasures. Thus, when a child is conceived, many will begin reading books aloud on the sciences or, perhaps, poetry. Beautiful music is played every day. Anything that can help the child to learn and grow in an advanced way—even before the child is born—is utilized. The time on earth is short, and these parents begin to work immediately to help make their child the best it can be. The point is so much time can be wasted on material and frivolous things. The soul is forever. Therefore, creative thought and the power of good (or bad) also go on forever.

Love is the ultimate achievement. No one would take the time to read this book if there is no interest in making a better life for the family. Love is the basis of all life. When it is withheld or denied, a person will fail to thrive. Self love is where it all begins. This isn't an ego trip where an individual's self esteem is so low that the attitude displayed is "I'm better than everyone else." It is an understanding within that a being of ultimate love, who is so great, beyond human imagination, created each soul. Therefore, each soul must honor itself as a treasure of this creation. Parents need to nurture this in themselves as well as their children. This is the only way that everything can change for the better.

It is common that human thoughts are negative. I, personally, refuse to be plagued with them. I use the words of Emile Coué to build subconscious power. These words chase those lower vibration thoughts away. Coué explained in his book how this tapping into the subconscious mind amazingly works. Everyone can do this. It is easy. The only cost is a bit of time, and the benefits are overwhelming. Those special words that have helped so many are the following:

Day by day,	Day by day,
in every way,	in every way,
I am getting	God is making me
better and better.	better and better.

People who do not trust or believe in themselves may need to change "I am getting" to "God is making me" better and better. Some have better success with this approach. If in doubt use both ways.

This little affirmation should be repeated 20 times when awakening and 20 times while preparing to sleep. Every child must learn this as early as possible. If a child is too small to say this affirmation, the mother or father can say positive words near the child while he/she is falling asleep or sleeping. What a change this planet would experience if all people did this.

Kids need care. What else in life is meaningful? When children are nourished physically, mentally, and spiritually, they thrive and flourish. Unfortunately, old destructive familial patterns are carried on from generation to generation. Nearly everyone has battle scars from childhood, but this cannot stop the forward thrust of a positive life. Give the child within permission to live in unconditional love. Then give every child in the family a rightful chance to grow in the light. Without light no flowers bloom.

Appendix A

Important News and Notes

Hangnails are a sign of folic acid deficiency. In infants deficiency of folic acid will cause spina bifida. Many primitive cultures always prepared the couple for pregnancy by insuring that the man and the woman had the best possible food, before, during, and after pregnancy. The resulting children were strong, healthy, and mentally bright as well as alert with no behavioral problems. Diet is probably the most important key for bearing bright, healthy, and happy kids. Isn't it somewhat arrogant that these wise and caring people are labeled as primitives?

According to Dr. Weston A. Price when the Eskimos ate only their wild natural forage, they had wide dental arches and strong beautiful teeth. When the Eskimo children were raised on the Standard American Diet, their dental arches were malformed and their teeth were crooked and full of caries (decay). After the children's parents changed their diets to processed food, the parents' teeth still appeared to be beautiful. However, upon examination one-third to two-thirds of their teeth were infected with dental caries. Thus, Dr. Price proved that dental caries are a sign of immune system deficiency. Further, a compromised immune system is due to poor nutrition from the Standard American Diet of refined, adulterated, and contaminated food.

According to the *American Journal of Epidemiology* the top 10 foods/drinks consumed by Americans are:

(1) white bread, rolls, crackers. White bread/cracker products are refined to such a degree that no nourishment is left, and only a small amount of synthetic vitamins are added back to what is virtually baked paste. Plus, they contain a number of chemicals and additives that the body cannot identify and utilize.

(2) doughnuts, cookies, cakes. Doughnuts, cookies, and cakes are the same white flour nightmare. However, they also contain a high amount of refined sugar and bad shortening (trans fats) or highly refined oils. These oils may be derived from genetically modified plants. Doughnuts are usually deep-fried in fat held at high temperatures. This fat is used repeatedly. This means that the structure of the overheated fat molecule breaks down, and it is oxidized and toxic.

(3) alcoholic beverages. Alcohol not only destroys millions of brain cells, but it also weakens cell membranes. This cellular weakening increases the risks for infection and cancer. Alcohol is a solvent, and certain types are made with GMOs. Children and, especially, females are severely damaged by consistent alcohol intake.

(4) commercial milk. Young girls who consume large quantities of commercial milk are developing breast cancer due to the contamination of milk with bovine growth hormone. Furthermore, boys are developing breasts.

(5) hamburgers, cheeseburgers, etc. Hamburgers and cheeseburgers and other fast foods are made with the cheapest resources available and lack virtually any nutritive value. They are full of the common contaminants, such as feces and chemical additives.

(6) beef steaks, roasts. Beef steaks and roasts are derived from potentially sick creatures that are raised or finished on GMO-tainted grains and pellets laced with animal remains. Cattle are supposed to be herbivores only. Then, as newspaper pictures have shown, if the pitiful animal can hobble into the slaughterhouse, it is horribly and painfully killed. The remains of the terrified, sick animals end up on dinner plates. That means at the very least that the meat is filled with adrenal hormones and toxic chemicals. This is passed on to the diner. Bon apétite.

(7) soft drinks. Soft drinks are known as soda, soda pop, pop, coke, tonic, or fizzy drinks throughout the world. This term may also include iced tea, lemonade, squash, and fruit punch. These drinks cause obesity. They provide empty calories with little to no food value.

There is also a relationship between a high consumption of these drinks and Type II diabetes. Furthermore, a high rate of tooth decay is prevalent in those who consume such drinks, which are sweetened with high fructose corn syrup, sugar, and glucose. Oral bacteria ferment these simple sugars. Acid is produced during this fermentation process. This acid dissolves tooth enamel. Thus, dental caries are a common result. Plus, some drinks are already acidic. Some have an acidic pH around 3.0 or even lower. Thus, the results are a physical disaster for the soft drink consumer.

Children who consume soft drinks daily may be ingesting high levels of caffeine. Caffeine frequently disrupts sleep. Thus, these children may have sleep disturbances and are often fatigued during the day.

Likewise, benzene as sodium benzoate is another chemical found in some soft drinks. This substance causes cancer. Benzoate may react with other additives, such as ascorbic acid or erythorbic acid, causing toxicity.

Aspartame is, yet, another story. The Douglass Report states that "aspartame is one of the most dangerous substances ever added to food." It is associated with such health problems as cancer, convulsions, lupus, and headaches. Brain tumors may develop, since it is a neurotoxin. Methanol poisoning is a common consequence. This poison is freely allowed in the marketplace, and children are among the biggest consumers of this deadly chemical. Plus, it actually is a cause of childhood obesity.

Bone density is also an issue. Children who break bones easily and fail to heal appropriately are frequently large consumers of soft drinks. Their body chemistries are awry. Usually, their diets needs to be altered as well as soft drink consumption must be omitted.

(8) hot dogs, ham, luncheon meats. Hot dogs, ham, luncheon meats are all processed meats, which contain many disgusting things. This includes guts, waste material, and nitrates and nitrites, the latter being carcinogens. Who knows what all is combined to make these processed concoctions. Many religions maintain pork is unfit for human consumption. Yet, it is the most common ingredient in processed meats.

(9) eggs. Eggs are healthy if the hens run free in the sunshine and eat the grass seeds, insects, greens, and all their natural forage. However, many are fed pellets made from feedlot entrails and other substances, which no living

creature should eat. The little pellets look so clean and neat. Yet, they are not the appropriate food for the creatures. Commercial egg production methods designate the feeding of such pellets. The chickens are also locked up in cages inside a building with no trace of sunshine, ever. Then, their eggs and tissues become food for people. The eggs and their tissues carry contaminants from the pellets and the environment as well. So much for the concept of the healing properties of chicken soup.

(10) French fries, potato chips. French fries and potato chips are, virtually, pillows of fat. Restaurants, hospitals, and schools use the potato to "clean" their hot grease. Many types of commercial French fries are made from potato powder and synthetic ingredients. One of these ingredients is propylene glycol, which is anti-freeze. Some contain no traces of potato at all. At a giant food show in Chicago there was a press for a powdered substance mixed with water. This made foot-long French fries to go with foot-long hot dogs. The man in the booth said it was a law that propylene glycol (anti-freeze) must be added to the French fry mixture. This requirement was to insure consistency and crunchiness of the finished product.

These are the top ten products consumed by Americans with just a small revelation of what they really are. There are thousands of so-called foods and drinks which provide nothing beneficial for the body. This is why the people and animals of the USA are fat and sick. When other nations adopt American ways, they also become fat and sick. Now, Australia has surpassed the United States for having the fattest citizens in the world.

Mercury may be found in various forms. Whether it is a vapor or an inorganic salt, it is highly poisonous. The first well-known adverse effect was on the brain. In the 1920s "mad as a hatter" became a well-known phrase. The top hat makers used mercury in their finishing processes. Besides brain damage, mercury injures the kidneys and lungs. It also activates many diseases and causes terrible birth defects.

Certain specific symptoms are regularly associated with mercury. These include vision, hearing, and speech impairment. Further, some may suffer a lack of coordination and peripheral neuropathy. In young children there may be neurological damage, and the myelin sheaths fail to form. Other symptoms include abnormally pink cheeks, fingertips, and toes as well as abnormally red lips. Swelling, itching, and skin peeling in layers are observed in some poisoned individuals. Additional symptoms include falling hair, loss of teeth and nails, rashes, muscle weakness, eye sensitivity to light, and memory loss. Profuse sweating, rapid heartbeat, high blood pressure, and excessive salivation are also triggered. So, don't poison your child with mercury-based amalgam fillings.

Chronic ear infections, tonsillitis, sore throats, and asthma are nearly always related to food allergies, which cause inflammation. These tissues are so weakened by allergenic foods that they readily become infected. Even healthy foods can cause allergy reactions. When the foods which cause the allergic reaction are eliminated the earaches, tonsillitis/sore throats, and wheezing are frequently eliminated as well.

A child's immune system is not well established until around age nine. So, until then allergy testing through blood testing is not appropriate. Just keep a chart of what the child has been eating, and see if there is a pattern to food allergy reactions. Also, kinesiology and/or pulse testing may be used to determine allergies.

Many food allergies are due to foods that an individual either loves or hates. At least that is a good starting place to determine what foods may be a problem. An individual may potentially react to a food for up to four days. That is why a rotation diet allows all food to be eaten only once every four days. If a reaction is obvious and repeated, it is best to eliminate the offending food completely from the diet. For further allergy solutions read Dr. Doris Rapp's book. She has been successful with desensitization of allergens.

Constant nose-picking indicates parasite infestation.

Frequent nose bleeds indicate a low calcium level.

Bed-wetting indicates fungus, gluten intolerance, allergies, and/or low blood sugar problems. This can be related to weak adrenal glands. Eliminate sugar and junk food. Use natural-source vitamin C, high grade 3x royal jelly, and B$_5$, the latter being known as pantothenic acid.

Thumb-sucking may be related to weak adrenal glands, since the adrenal glands are the coping mechanism of the body. This behavior is comforting for the stressed child. Some take action against the child for this habit. If it is merely gently removing the thumb from a baby's mouth, it is not a problem. However, spanking, using substances that burn the mouth, and other harsh methods will only stress the child further. Again, eliminating the junk and sugar from the diet is important. Supplement the diet with high B complex foods, plus, natural vitamin C, high grade royal jelly/bee pollen, and raw purple maca drops.

Craving something sweet, then something salty, then something sweet, and then something salty is a definite sign of adrenal weakness. The individual needs support with the appropriate diet and additional nutritional support as mentioned above.

Coarse hair is a sign of thyroid weakness. This person needs extra thyroid support. The diet should be free of goitrogenic foods such as raw cabbage, raw Brussel sprouts, raw carrots, raw flax, raw peanuts, raw cashews, and raw strawberries. Yet, a special type of kelp called bull kelp is beneficial, especially when combined with wild oregano and the amino acid tyrosine.

Baby fine hair indicates a super sensitive system, and this individual will need less food and smaller dosages of supplements. Only the finest quality food and supplements should be used with this extremely sensitive person.

Excessive hair loss is usually related to impaired thyroid function.

Pain behind the left eye is a sign of pituitary swelling or impairment.

When headaches occur frequently, the individual has significant food allergies. Any individual who suffers from frequent severe headaches can find relief by determining the food allergies and eliminating those foods from the diet. Wild raw liquid green herbal drops rich in B_2 are usually beneficial, when a headache does occur. These wild greens drops include dandelion leaves, burdock, and nettles, which help detoxify the liver.

Headaches begin in the gut. Treat the gut, and the headaches will cease. Digestive enzymes, certain spices, and Super-5 Greens juice are frequently helpful. The wild, raw tripple green drops previously mentioned are especially helpful in reversing digestive headaches.

Children who smell bad even after a good scrubbing are deficient in calcium, magnesium, and zinc.

Constipation is one of the most common problems among children. It is mainly caused by poor eating and drinking habits. A deficiency of thiamine and other B vitamins is especially significant. A few schools have eliminated the synthetic drink and junk food machines. Some schools are making an effort to provide healthy, even organic, food for the students. The difference in health and behavior among the students is beyond significant.

According to Dr. Jorgen Clausen, a Danish biochemist, multiple sclerosis is associated with unsaturated fatty acid deficiency. Likewise, it was determined that bottle-fed babies have a higher occurrence of MS than breast-fed babies. Additionally, aspartame may be a factor.

According to Suzine Stockton, investigative reporter, the toxicity of industrial fluoride is vast. Based on a number of studies this noxious chemical can cause a wide range of disorders, including hyperactivity, lowered IQ, birth defects, Down's syndrome, early onset puberty, interference with the pineal gland (the producer of melatonin), Alzheimer's disease, hypothyroidism, genetic mutations, cancer, immune system defects, increased rates of hip fractures in older people, infertility, and gastrointestinal problems.

Many parents don't realize that children worry. Many children do worry and are unhappy. Some are lonely and without friends. All these children are sick more frequently than children who have no such problems. They may fall into bad patterns such as drinking alcohol, drug abuse, and other self-destructive behaviors. Often, they are a reflection of adult behavior around them. At a minimum they are, no doubt, nutritionally depleted.

Wild food and herbs taken from a non-polluted area are more powerful and nutritious than even organic food. Learn about these plants, berries, and herbs. Organize a family outing to find and pick them. Make use of them as soon after picking as possible, because the powerful photonic energy and nutrients are soon depleted. You will see and feel the difference. Besides, the sunshine, fresh air, and family comradery will be highly beneficial as well.

Slow Food is an organization which began in Italy. Carlo Petrini formed a group of small farmers who wanted to supply beautiful, wholesome food to all interested parties. Now, this worthy organization has spread worldwide. These small farmers usually employ natural farming techniques. Most use heirloom seeds to produce superb plants and beautiful food. Some raise rare breeds of poultry and animals. Others provide wild fish products. The worldwide assault by agribusiness has made it difficult if not impossible for small farmers to survive. Thus, the most delicious and wholesome food in the world was quickly disappearing. All the food produced on these small farms may not be certified organic. This is because of the cost and huge amount of paperwork required for certification. However, most farms are not using chemicals and poisons or are in transition.

The Slow Food show each year has booths where the farmers and small manufacturers bring their wares. To say that it is some of the best food I have ever eaten is a bit of an understatement. I wanted to bring all of the products into the United States. Unfortunately, the paperwork and excessive import fees of around $1500 per item make it difficult to do so. However, the small farmers in the United States are joining this organization and are beginning to supply lovely, unadulterated, chemical free food as well. Look up Slow Food on the internet, and become a member. Be kind to yourself, and always eat truly delicious, healthy food.

Some think organic food is too expensive. Yet, it is way too expensive not to eat the very best food, either home grown or purchased. Personal health and the health of every family member is the most valuable possession. Without good health life is even a greater challenge than it normally is.

Try growing something, maybe a favorite food or herbs, for example. If there is no yard available, use containers. Kids love to see the miracle of life that develops from a single seed. Sunshine, seeds, healthy fertile soil, and water are the only requirements. The return for a little work is many fold. It will provide the household with fresh produce that will nourish the body and the soul.

In Germany a window is open year-round in the home, especially wherever the toilet is located. Fresh air/oxygen is mandatory for the body to function as it should.

Cities do not adequately purify their water. Water towers have been found to contain dead animals. Huge amounts of chlorine and other deadly chemicals are added to water supplies, so that diseases such as cholera do not occur. However, the human body is mostly water, and that is why water quality is so important. Public drinking water contains far more than the natural minerals, which are healthy. As a whole the general public is popping four or more medications daily. What happens to that medication? It is excreted as urine or feces into the public sewers, which drain into the lakes, streams, and aquifers. Ultimately, everyone is drinking and showering in someone else's drug waste material. The body will absorb more chemicals and drug waste through showering and bathing than drinking eight glasses of water a day. Small children love to play in the bathtub for extended periods of time. Although children should be supervised while bathing, the biggest danger to them is not necessarily drowning. The major danger is absorbing all the toxic substances in the water. This is a huge health threat. Deformities of fish and water creatures are at an all time high. Men in some very toxic areas are growing breasts. Some areas have direly high cancer incidences. The powerful cardiovascular drugs should not be in the bodies of small children and in those who have no cardiovascular problems. Too many people are on mind-altering drugs as well. These drugs change the personality and demeanor and not necessarily for the better. Water filtration for drinking and bathing is a must in this extremely polluted world.

Children not much older than toddlers are using cell phones and computers. There is absolute evidence that shows cell phones cause brain disruption. These devices are quite capable of activating tumor growth at any age. A 10-year study links four kinds of cancer to cell phone use. Children and adults for that matter do not need to be glued to a cell phone engaged in useless chatter. At best a cell phone should be used for emergencies only.

When a person attempts to do something and repeatedly fails to accomplish the goal, something has to change. No one can expect to repeat the same behavior or activity over and over, and then get different results. Thus, if reactions are the same from many people, or you expect to have tea and it's always coffee, check yourself first. For example, if people are always taking advantage of you, it is because you are doing something that allows them to do so. If you want tea, don't use coffee in the pot. You must change the behavior—or the beverage—to get different results.

It is interesting to note that a book dated 1921 explains that children should be fed "real, old-fashioned foods." It says that "plain coarse food is needed. Sandwiches are permissible, but the bread should be coarse (whole grain) and kept free of spiced meats and bologna (processed meats). Fried foods should be avoided, and fried steak never included." It is not a new idea that processed foods are of little value. The less informed people are about healthy food, the more sophisticated they think refined, lifeless food really is. Of course, the advertisements are very compelling. The Mexican people as they moved into the United States, became addicted to all the brightly packaged refined junk food. Now each generation is experiencing a decline. Their babies are not so strong and active. The parents don't have the energy to do what their parents did. It is a living experiment in action, and few are watching and learning.

In the same 1921 book it has a section on boiled vegetables. For example, the directions for preparing asparagus was to boil for 20 to 25 minutes. Beets were to be boiled for four to six hours. Did these people have teeth, or did they like to drink vegetable slime? Now we know that raw food is almost always preferable to cooked food. If food is cooked, it should be as briefly as possible. The nutrients and enzymes are vitally important. They are lost with prolonged cooking over high heat in lots of liquid.

Appendix B

RELIGIOUS EXEMPTION FROM VACCINATION

DATE _____

I _____,

claim religious exemption under section 167.181 RSMO due to religious and moral convictions. My objections are listed below as follows:

Public Law 97-280, passed by the 97th Congress of the United States of America, declares the Bible to Be the "Word of God" and directs citizens to "study and apply the teachings of the Holy Scriptures. The Bible teaches that the truthfulness of an issue is to be sought and should stand on no less than two or more witnesses." (Deuteronomy 19:15)

A diligent search for truth on the safety and effectiveness of vaccinations reveals there are many studied, informed and qualified witnesses who have found and teach that there are serious health risks involved with vaccinations. Even Senate Bill 732 before the 103rd Congress of the United States, known as the "Comprehensive Child Health Immunization Act of 1993," makes known the fact that there are risks to vaccines. The following words are from that bill: "Vaccine information materials should be simplified to ensure that parents can understand the *benefits and risks* of vaccines" (emphasis added).

The Bible teaches that there are clean and unclean animals and that God's people are not to put the unclean into their bodies (Deuteronomy 14). Furthermore, the Bible teaches that "Ye shall not eat of anything that dieth of itself" (Deuteronomy 14:21) and "that flesh with the life thereof, which is the blood thereof, shall ye not eat." (Genesis 9:4) Vaccines are often made of, or embody, fetuses or eggs of said unclean creatures. The process of creating the vaccine often causes said creatures to die in the process (i.e., dieth of itself). Many vaccines are made in or of the blood of diseased animals.

"What? know ye not that your body is the temple of the Holy Ghost which is in you, which ye have of God, and ye are not your own. For ye are bought with a price: therefore glorify God in your body, and in your spirit, which are God's." (I Corinthians 6:19, 20)

The Bible teaches that we are not to harm or wrong our neighbor. (Romans 13:10: James 2:8) Our decision to decline vaccinations does not wrong or threaten our neighbor. If vaccinations are truly effective, then vaccinated neighbors would be in no danger from someone who is not vaccinated. Also, statistics show that those NOT vaccinated are less likely to expose their neighbor to harmful pathogens (that are contained in the vaccinations).

Hepatitis B Not Highly Contagious—unlike other infectious diseases for which vaccines have been developed and mandated in the U.S., hepatitis B is not common in childhood and is not highly contagious. Hepatitis B is primarily an adult disease transmitted through infected body fluids, most frequently infected blood, and is prevalent in high risk populations such as needle-using drug addicts, sexually promiscuous heterosexual and homosexual adults, residents and staff of custodial institutions such as prisons, health care workers exposed to blood, persons who require repeated blood transfusions and babies born to infected mothers.

According to *CDC Prevention Guidelines: A Guide to Action* (1997), a book written by federal public health officials at the U.S. government centers for Disease Control (CDC), "the sources of [hepatitis B] infection for most cases include intravenous drug use (28%) heterosexual contact with infected persons or multiple partners (22%) and homosexual activity (9%)." According to *Harrison's Principles of Internal Medicine* (1944), mother-to-child transmission of hepatitis B "is common in North America and western Europe.

Although CDC officials have made statements that hepatitis B is easy to catch through sharing toothbrushes or razors, Eric Mast, M.D., Chief of the Surveillance Section, Hepatitis Branch of the CDC, stated in a 1997 public hearing that: "although [the hepatitis B virus] is present in moderate concentrations in saliva, it's not transmitted commonly by casual contact."

Some of the ingredients of our current vaccines are:
(1) **formaldehyde**, used in production of resins, plastics, and foam insulation, and as a preservative, disinfectant, and antibacterial food additive. It is a known carcinogen (can initiate a new cancer), commonly used to embalm corpses.

(2) **Thimerosal**, a mercury derivative. The heavy metal mercury is toxic to the central nervous system and not easily eliminated from the body. "Aluminum, formaldehyde and mercury"—including the mercury in "silver" dental fillings and amalgams (see Chapter 9)—"have a long history of documented hazardous effects including cancer, neurological damage" such as multiple sclerosis, Lou Gehrig's disease, "and death."

Studies report, "Thimerosal inhibits phagocytes, one of the body's most vital immune defenses in blood." Then what effect will it have on healthy human cells after it is injected into the bloodstream? Jamie Murphy, a concerned nonprofessional observer asks, "Who would take chemicals that are carcinogenic in rats, are used in the manufacture of inks, dyes, explosives, wrinkle-proof fabrics, home insulation, and embalming fluid—and inject them into the delicate body of a baby?"

Among other vaccine ingredients are **aluminum phosphate**, **aluminum adjuvants**, **alum, and acetone**; **phenol** is included in allergy injections. "Benzoic acid, a preservative whose injection into rats causes tremors, convulsions, and death, is added. And then vaccine makers add decomposing animal proteins, such as pig or horse blood, cow pox pus, rabbit brain tissue, duck egg protein, and dog kidney tissue."

A glance at further steps in vaccine making is no less disturbing. To produce a "live" virus vaccine, such as MMR (measles/mumps/rubella), the virus is passed through animal tissue several times to reduce its potency. **Measles virus is passed through chick embryos, polio virus through monkey kidney, and the rubella virus is passed through the dissected organs of an aborted human fetus.**

"Killed' vaccines are 'inactivated' through heat, radiation, or chemicals. The weakened germ is then strengthened with antibody boosters and stabilizers. This is done by the addition of **drugs**, **antibiotics** and **toxic**

disinfectants: neomycin, streptomycin, sodium chloride, sodium hydroxide, aluminum hydroxide, aluminum hydrochloride, sorbitol, hydrolyzed gelatin, formaldehyde [again], and thimerosal [again]."

Injected straight into the child's bloodstream—bypassing the cellular immune system, one-half of our protective immunity mechanism, those materials destroy stores of protective nutrients in the tiny body. So it is not hard to see why epidemic vaccines worsen health throughout life.

Only two single-antigen pediatric hepatitis B vaccines exist on the US market, Engerix-B (SmithKline Beecham) and Recombivax HB (Merck). Both contain thimerosal and 12.5 micrograms of mercury per 0.5 ml dose.

Bibliography

Adams, Ruth and Murray, Frank. 1972. *Body, Mind and the B Vitamins.* New York, NY: Larchmont Books.

Airola, Paavo O. 1970. *Health Secrets from Europe.* West Nyack, NY: Parker Publishing Company.

Anderson, Kenneth N., Editor. 1994. *Mosby's Medical, Nursing, and Allied Health Dictionary.* St. Louis, MO: Mosby.

Barkie, Karen E. 1982. *Sweet and Sugarfree.* New York, NY: St. Martin's Press.

Benowicz, Robert J. 1981. *Vitamins and You.* New York, NY: A Berkley Book.

Bicknell, Franklin and Prescott, Frederick. 1953. *The Vitamins in Medicine.* London, England: William Heinemann Ltd.

Campbell, Susan and Winant, Todd. 1994. *Healthy School Lunch Action Guide.* Santa Cruz, CA: EarthSave Foundation.

Cooper, Lenna F., Barber, Edith M., Mitchell, Helen S.. 1947. *Nutrition in Health and Disease.* Philadelphia, PA: J. B. Lippincott Company.

Davis, Adelle. l965. *Let's Get Well.* New York, NY: The New American Library, Inc.

Eastwood, Martin. 1997. *Principles of Human Nutrition.* London, Weinheim, New York, Tokyo, Melbourne, Madras: Chapman and Hall.

Editorial Committee. 1973. *The Vitamins Explained Simply.* Melbourne, Victoria: Science of Life Books Pty. Ltd.

Elkington, John. 1986. *The Poisoned Womb.* Middlesex, England: Penguin Books Ltd.

Faelten, Sharon and the editors of Prevention Magazine. 1981. *The Complete Book of Minerals for Health.* Emmaus, Pennsylvania: Rodale Press.

French, William Fleming. 1921. *Your Children's Food*. by Calumet baking powder.

Grodner, Michele, Anderson, Sara Long, DeYoung, Sandra. 2000. Second Edition, *Foundations and Clinical Applications of Nutrition, A Nursing Approach*. St Louis, London, Toronto: Mosby.

Ingram, Cass. 1997. *The Cure is in the Cupboard*. Buffalo Grove, IL: Knowledge House Publishers.

Ingram, Cass. 1998. *Super-market Remedies*. Buffalo Grove, IL: Knowledge House Publishers.

Ingram, Cass. 2003. *The Longevity Solution*. Buffalo Grove, IL: Knowledge House Publishers.

Ingram, Cass. 2003. *The Respiratory Solution*. Buffalo Grove, IL: Knowledge House Publishers.

Ingram, Cass. 2005. *How to Eat Right and Live Longer*. Buffalo Grove, IL: Knowledge House Publishers.

Ingram, Cass. 2005. *Natural Cures for High Blood Pressure*. Buffalo Grove, IL: Knowledge House Publishers.

Ingram, Cass. 2005. *Natural Cures for Killer Germs*. Buffalo Grove, IL: Knowledge House Publishers.

Jacobi, Dana and the editors of Natural Health Magazine. 1995. *The Natural Health Cookbook*. New York, New York: Simon and Schuster.

Krause, Marie V. 1966. *Food, Nutrition and Diet Therapy*. Philadelphia, PA: W. B. Saunders Company.

Kirschmann, John D., with Dunne, Lavon J. 1984. Second Edition, *Nutrition Almanac*. New York, London, Toronto: McGraw-Hill Book Company.

Kugelmass, L. Newton. 1942. *Superior Children Through Modern Nutrition*. New York, N Y: E. P. Dutton and Co., Inc.

Lieberman, Shari and Bruning, Nancy. 1990. *The Real Vitamin & Mineral Book*. Garden City Park, NY: Avery Publishing Group.

Longgood, William. 1960. *The Poisons in Your Food*. New York, NY: Simon and Schuster.

Mathews, Albert P. 1937. *Vitamins, Minerals and Hormones*. Baltimore, MD: William Wood and Company.

McGill, Marion and Pye, Orrea. 1978. *The No-Nonsense Guide to Food and Nutrition*. New York, NY: Butterick Publishing.

Mitchell, Rynbergen, Anderson, Dibble. 1968. *Cooper's Nutrition in Health and Disease*. Philadelphia, PA: J. B. Lippincott Company.

Pattee, Alida Frances. 1943. *Vitamins and Minerals For Everyone*. New York, NY: Putnam's Sons.

Price, Westin A. 2006. *Nutrition and Physical Degeneration*. 7th Edition. La Mesa, CA: The Price-Pottenger Nutrition Foundation, Inc.

Quesnell, William R. 2000. *Minerals The Essential Link to Health*. La Mesa, CA: Skills Unlimited Press.

Quillin, Patrick. 1989. *Healing Nutrients*. New York: Vintage Books.

Robertson, Laurel, Carol Flinders, and Brian Ruppenthal. 1986. *The New Laurel's Kitchen*. Berkley, California: Ten Speed Press.

Satter, Ellyn. 1987. *How to Get Your Kid to Eat*. Palo Alto, CA: Bull Publishing Company.

Schmidt, Michael A. 1996. *Healing Childhood Ear Infections*. Berkley, CA: North Atlantic Books.

Sherman, Henry C. 1937. *Chemistry of Food and Nutrition*. New York, NY: The Macmillan Company.

Sherman, Henry C. 1947. *Food and Health*. New York, NY: The Macmillan Company.

Smith, Lendon. 1979. *Feed Your Children Right*. New York, NY: McGraw-Hill Book Company.

Smith, Vearl R. 1966. *Physiology of Lactation*. Ames, IA: Iowa State University Press.

Wachter, Kerri. January 2010. *Complimentary Foods Move Beyond Rice Cereal.* pps. 70-71. Rockville, MD. Family Practice News.

Wade, Carlson. 1967. *Magic Minerals, Key to Better Health.* West Nyack, NY: Parker Publishing Company, Inc.

Wade, Carlson. 1972. *Vitamins and Other Food Supplements and Your Health.* New Canaan, CT: Keats Publishing, Inc.

Wade, Carlson. 1975. *Miracle Protein: Secret of Natural Cell-Tissue Rejuvenation.* West Nyack, NY: Parker Publishing Company, Inc.

Williams, Dr. Roger J. 1978. *Nutrition Against Disease.* New York, NY: Pitman Publishing Company.

Williams, Sue Rodwell. 1969. *Nutrition and Diet Therapy.* St. Louis, MO: The C. V. Mosby Company.

Winick, Myron, Editor. 1972. *Nutrition and Development.* New York, NY: John Wiley & Sons.

Index

deficiency signs and symptoms,
178
functions of, 177-178
source of and requirements for,
178-179
Vitamin K, 164, 180-181

W

Wade, Carlson, 186
Whipped Cream Topping, 284
White and Green Salad, 273
Why We Are What We Are, 300
Wolback, Dr., 158

X

X-rays, 62-63

Y

Yeast, 52, 97, 105-106, 111, 113, 116,
121, 123, 135-137, 139, 179, 212

Z

Zinc, 54, 66, 160, 188, 206-210, 314
functions of, 206-208
deficiency of, 206-208
sources of, 208